ALLOWING THE DESTRUCTION OF LIFE UNWORTHY OF LIFE.

ITS MEASURE AND FORM.

by

Jurist and Law Professor Karl Binding, PhD.
University of Leipzig.

Doctor and Medical Professor Alfred Hoche, M.D.
University of Freiburg.

Originally Published in 1920

Translated by Dr. Cristina Modak

Commissioned by the Policy Intersections Research Center
www.policyintersections.org

Published by

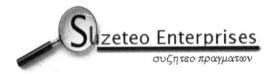

Suzeteo Enterprises
συζητεο πραγματων

ALLOWING THE DESTRUCTION OF LIFE UNWORTHY OF LIFE.

ITS MEASURE AND FORM.

by

Jurist and Law Professor Karl Binding, PhD.
University of Leipzig.

Doctor and Medical Professor Alfred Hoche, M.D.
University of Freiburg.

Originally Published in 1920

Translated by Dr. Cristina Modak

Commissioned by the Policy Intersections Research Center
www.policyintersections.org

Published by

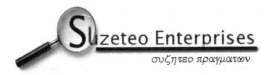

Suzeteo Enterprises
συζητεο πραγματων

Allowing the Destruction of Life Unworthy of Life
by Karl Binding and Alfred Hoche

Translated by Dr. Cristina Modak.

Translation commissioned by the
Policy Intersections Research Center
www.policyintersections.org

Foreword by PIRC Director, Dr. Anthony Horvath.

Soft Cover ISBN 978-1-936830-50-3
Hard Cover ISBN 978-1-936830-75-6
Ebook ISBN 978-1-936830-51-0

Official Website for the Book: www.lifeunworthyoflife.com

A Note on the Text:

The translation is based on the text that was best available to the translator and publisher. Sections in brackets [...] indicate words not explicitly in the original German but required in the English to properly convey the meaning of the text. The original German text is provided at the end of this document.

Foreword

1. Prelude

In the minds of many moderns, the horrors of the 20th century represent far off events wholly detached from our present understanding of the world. They belong in the same mental compartment as the destruction of Jerusalem in 70 AD or the barbarian pillages of Rome. As an icon of evil, Hitler is roughly in the same category as Attila the Hun, representing an extreme and singular perturbation of history, appearing without cause and having no effects, and certainly having no relevance to the present day.

As of this writing, however, the 20th century concluded just about a decade ago. Let that sink in. It was *not* some far off event. It was practically just yesterday. The Third Reich toppled down ignominiously, even if drenched in the blood of millions, just seventy years ago. This will be within the lifetime of many readers. There may even be those alive who remember it; certainly, there are still many who heard of it not in history books, but from the mouths of parents and grandparents, from those who endured it first-hand, and may indeed have helped bring it down.

Perhaps because of its staggering scale, there is reluctance to look upon the last century with the kind of scrutiny it requires, yet it is precisely because of that scale that we must make sure that we learn from it. To begin with, we must face up to the fact that the atrocities of the 20th century did *not* spring up out of the universe as historical accidents. They followed from particular events in human history that paralleled the emergence and dominance of particular philosophies. Some of these philosophies have become wide-spread, and even dominant, once again.

The bloodbath that was the 20th century *did* have causes and contributing factors. The book you have in your hand right now is one of them, but modern readers may have trouble fathoming why on earth that should be the case. Except for some occasionally jarring language to our modern sensibilities, most of Binding and Hoche's arguments are within the mainstream of today's 'ethical' thought.

And what is there to object to? After all, can't we all agree that a person facing a future of perpetual, intense suffering, is facing a life that is not worth living? Only a heartless and cruel person could possibly stand in the way of allowing that person a quiet, dignified, and humane release. Right? On top of that, considering the fact that there are scarce medical resources available, society has a duty and obligation to ensure that those resources are allocated towards those who can expect a good quality of life. *Right?*

Perhaps the reader doesn't appreciate that characterization of the issue, but it is in fact the kind of language and argumentation being advanced in health care today. Documenting it is outside the scope of this essay, but for a treatment specifically on the topic, turn to Wesley J. Smith's *Culture of Death: The Assault on Medical Ethics in America*. It has an entire chapter titled "Life Unworthy of Life" that draws the connection making specific reference to the present book by Binding and Hoche.

The purpose of this essay is different.

Not everyone finds the information that Mr. Smith has documented to be all that disconcerting—obviously, since there must be people out there actually saying and doing those things in order for him to document them. Indeed, many find the ideas more or less acceptable. That these ideas were latched onto by the National Socialists is unfortunate, but that doesn't necessarily discredit them, does it? Those ideas don't necessarily have to lead to a holocaust, do they?

For the purpose of this essay, we will suppose that such a thing is hypothetically possible, but it must be strongly stated that if that is to be the case, then it can only be the case if the *right* lessons are actually drawn from recent history. Sadly, lessons have been drawn, but they are the *wrong* ones. Delving deep into what the right lessons might be is also not the purpose of this essay.

To *even begin* drawing the right lessons, we have to ask ourselves *how* it was that something as 'innocuous' as Binding and Hoche's *Allowing the Destruction of Life Unworthy of Life* could serve as a catalyst for some of humanity's worst atrocities. There are reasons why that was the case, and it is to some of those reasons we turn to now. The rest is up to the reader.

2. *Res ipsa loquitur*

Religion is an insult to human dignity. With or without
it you would have good people doing good things and
evil people doing evil things. But for good people to do
evil things, that takes religion.

Few statements illustrate the human inclination towards self-
deception as this one by physicist Steven Weinberg. If anything,
if one were to make an honest assessment from *actual* history,
the correct rendition would be "for good people to do evil
things, that takes *science*."

Few people today realize that the Nazis, communists, fasc-
ists, and Marxists that carried out the atrocities of the 20th century all believed that A., they were good people and B., they
were acting on *scientific* principles. Insofar as this is recognized
today, their schemes and operating principles are now regarded
as 'pseudo-scientific.'

Naturally, the people at the time did not view it as *pseudo* at
all. Whether or not present day attitudes on what we regard as
'scientific' will be labeled as 'pseudo-scientific' in fifty years remains to be seen. Fish do not know they are wet.

Claims that the scientific views of these people were actually
'pseudo-science' usually comes without any analysis of what, in
particular, made it *pseudo*. After all, many of those views are in
circulation today.

As a case in point, consider the argument put forward by
modern (and avowed) eugenicist, Julian Savulescu, the editor of
journal on medical ethics. In a *Reader's Digest* article, he wrote:

Much of the unease about designer babies comes from
the work of the 20th-century eugenics movement. It
tried to use selective breeding to weed out criminals, the
insane and the poor, based on the false belief that such
conditions were caused *only* by genetic disorders. It
reached its inglorious climax when the Nazis moved
beyond sterilisation to exterminate the "genetically unfit". [emphasis mine]

I emphasized the word 'only' to ask this question: "And so, *if*
their belief *had been accurate*, and criminals, the insane and the

poor, were *in fact* caused *only* by genetic disorders, would *that* have made the Nazi effort proper and justified?"[1]

One comes away from Savulescu's dismissal of the Nazi horror as less-than-scientific without being greatly comforted: his argument seems to be more or less the same. He only requires better information—a more scientific basis for his 'selective breeding.'

Savulescu distinguishes his proposals from that of the Nazis because he is calling for voluntary action. He places the moral obligation to 'select ethically better children' on the shoulders of parents, not the state. Obviously, though, if the parents are *morally* obligated to do this, then society is *morally* obligated to consider what to do if parents don't make the 'right' decision. *Shouldn't* society intervene? Savulescu does not say in this article, but Binding and Hoche have a ready answer, as you will see.

One underlying premise shared by all three men is that the mere knowing of the right facts give us self-evident moral guidance on what to do with those facts. On Savulescu's presentation, if we know our child will have "dispositions to violence"[2] then it is self-evident that the parent should discard that one in favor of one without that genetic disposition. He asks:

> Surely trying to ensure that your children have the best, or a good enough, opportunity for a great life is responsible parenting? If we have the power to intervene in the nature of our offspring—rather than consigning them to the natural lottery—then we should.

"National Socialism is nothing but applied biology," said Nazi thug, Rudolf Hess, but as you can see, that is all Savulescu is doing, too. He says, "If it were possible to genetically select good impulse control, we should do so." And, "...the future of humanity is in our hands now. Rather than fearing genetics, we should embrace it."

---

[1] Ironically, Savulescu goes on to advocate for selective breeding for psychological traits that he implies *only* have a genetic basis, "such as potential alcoholism, psychopathy and dispositions to violence." He says: "[Y]ou could argue that people have a moral obligation to select ethically better children."

[2] For example. You can insert any physical characteristic or behavior presumed to be 'bad.' Note how many times he uses the word 'should.'

Savulescu and Hess agree that if we know something about biology, we *should* act on that knowledge. They both seem to believe that the biological 'facts on the ground' lend themselves to *res ipsa loquitur*, "the thing speaks for itself." Further, the knowledge itself points us in the right direction for what to do with that knowledge. The two differ on the nature of the thing, so their application of the biology will differ somewhat, but the core premise remains intact:

> Whatever we conclude about the nature of humans and particular humans has implications that 'speak for themselves.' *And these implications are based on science, and acting on science is always good, and we* should *act.*

In framing it in this way, we now have a glimpse into how Binding and Hoche's work could have morphed into the horrors that it did. When one is talking poppycock about religion and ethics, one is in the domain of mere opinion. When one is talking about science, one is talking about the world as it really is. It is not the sort of thing to get squeamish about.[3]

Binding begins his part of the essay by saying, "The scientific clarification of the pertinent starting point is however so essential..." He believes he is proceeding along scientific lines as he reconciles German law with the propriety of destroying an 'unworthy life.'

He goes out of his way to dispense with religious rationale, which has no place in secular society. He specifically targets Christianity, labeling the Church's refusal to let people die 'good deaths' as unchristian. Binding believes he is standing on the firm ground of scientific reality: "I can find absolutely no reason, from a legal, social, moral, religious point of view, not to allow those that want it, to kill those beyond salvation, who desperately desire it."

Indeed, he believes that *his* is the compassionate view, saying that it stems "from the deepest compassion."

Or, to put it another way, given what he knows about compassion, and what he knows about people, allowing people to kill themselves is self-evidently the proper position for a scien-

---

[3] Savulescu says that the refusal to engage in rational selection "is to consign those who come after us to the ball and chain of our squeamishness and irrationality."

tifically minded person exhibiting "cool calculated logic."[4]

In large part, it is this notion *that certain conclusions follow self-evidently from scientific 'truths'* that lies behind the 20th century global eugenics movement. The same notion drove on the Marxists and the Nazis. The same unspoken presumption is with us today, unnoticed, and therefore not repudiated.

Clearly, though, that notion is not enough to get us from this document to the Holocaust.

3. Fact, Not Opinion

Let's take it from a different angle. Today, when the Nazis are remembered they are remembered as being fierce racists. Their anti-semitism, of course, is well known, but they also despised black people, gypsies, and pretty much anyone that did not have blond hair and blue eyes. Their despising was not of the visceral, sentimental sort. It was the cool, dispassionate, scientific sort; these despised groups of people reflected deficiencies within the human species that were continuing to propagate and pollute 'good stock.'

To understand how even-handed the Nazis were in this out-look, it is important to recall that before there were extermination camps, there was the T4 program. In the T4 program, disabled *Germans* of all ages were rounded up and quietly gassed. Read that again: *these were Germans.* Even former German war heroes were not safe from Germany's public 'health' policies—for that is what they were seen as: public health policies.[5]

The racial component is important in understanding the Holocaust but it cannot be seen as the root cause. After all, Binding and Hoche wrote this book before the Nazi party even existed, let alone took power. The ethical justification for euthanasia that they laid out was based on medical and scientific grounds, not racial ones. For the Nazis, the ethical basis for euthanizing disabled people was the same as the basis for euthanizing the Jews, which accounts for their even-handed destruction of their

---

[4] See page 16.

[5] Daniel Kevles explains how the Nazi eugenic movement, which was similar in many respects to the one in America and even applauded there, ran independently from its Anti-Semitism throughout the 1930s. See pages 116-119 of his *In the Name of Eugenics* (1995) for more.

fellow Germans before concluding that the Jews were also a drag on the *Volk*.[6]

To understand how Binding and Hoche's work could be put into service in this way, we must put their work into a greater context. For that, it is necessary to at least make mention of the so-called "Age of Enlightenment."

In Germany, this culminated with Nietzsche's proclamation that 'God was dead.' No longer held back by "religious beliefs, sentimental feelings and so on," the Germans, as with like-minded individuals in the United States and elsewhere in Europe, citizens were busily constructing new moralities based on new scientific facts. The 1800s was a century of optimism.

However, there was a difference between the attitudes and approaches espoused by those in the first half of the 1800s compared to those espoused in the second half. In the first five decades or so, Thomas Malthus's argument that human conflict was the result of overpopulation competing for scarce natural resources led to various ruminations about how to handle that 'problem.'[7]

Much of this talk was aimed at the poor, and the poor often were of different ethnicity than the people offering their proposals. One had their prejudice, but there it sat, as mere prejudice. One could not re-order society around it because one could not present it as anything more than "one man's opinion."[8]

Then came Charles Darwin in 1859 who, in his *On the Origin of Species by Means of Natural Selection, or the Preservation of Favoured Races in the Struggle for Life* ended the dispute decisively, putting one set of opinions on the firm foundation of

---

[6] In this context, the 'Volk' refers to the Nazi concept of the German people as a whole as an actual organism, which must be kept 'pure.'

[7] Not that Malthus was the first to put the notion out there. Jonathan Swift's 1729 *A Modest Proposal*, which (satirically) suggested that poor Irish people solve their economic problems by selling their children off as food, was a response to other kinds of proposals then common, which he felt were just as evil and absurd.

[8] Then there was the opposite view of the Church, which held that all people were made in the image of God, with their own intrinsic value. But religion consists exclusively of opinions, and have even less authority than opinions normally do. Still, whether it is the idea that humans are made in the image of God that they are animals, they are just ideas that some people hold. They are not weighty enough to force your fellowman to fall in line with them.

scientific fact—the Malthusian outlook—and *disproving* the religious one.[9] At least, that was how it was instantly perceived—and is still perceived to this day.

Darwin's evolutionary theory soon was firmly accepted within the scientific establishment and the implications were instantly grasped and acted on. Men like Francis Galton began openly discussing the need for 'eugenics' programs of various kinds.[10] In America, these and other proposals took on additional impetus due to the abolition of slavery after the civil war. Hundreds of thousands of freed slaves began to gravitate to the cities. Unable to fend for themselves, they were taxing public resources. They were ignorant, illiterate, feeble-minded idiots that *obviously* were biologically inferior compared to those of northern European stock.

After Darwin, the prejudice and racism that had previously existed as mere sentiment became something new: *scientific* racism. It was now grounded in reality, as proved by science. Now it was possible to take actions based on the absolute conviction that one was not merely playing to their own sensitivities, but rather were acting in view of cold, hard, scientific fact. And if anyone had any doubts, they needed only look to the newly emancipated negroes; nothing better illustrated the importance of quick and decisive application of biological principles.

The establishment of Darwinism as *a fact* by anyone with half a brain brought with it two important ramifications that sprung up at the same time and in the same strength. On the one hand, the philosophical question about whether or not humans were just another kind of animal was now answered definitively

---

[9] Darwin actually credits Malthus as being an important influence on his thinking. What Darwin added to the Malthusian outlook was the idea that in the competition for scarce resources, some parts of the population would die, leaving only the stronger parts. In this way, death was actually a vehicle by which a population was improved. 'Natural Selection' was a *creative* power; indeed, it was the explanation for how all life came to be.

[10] It was Galton, Darwin's cousin, who coined the word 'eugenics' in 1883. He thought that Eugenics "must be introduced into the national conscience, like a new religion. It has, indeed, strong claims to become an orthodox religious, tenet of the future, for eugenics co-operate with the workings of nature by securing that humanity shall be represented by the fittest races. What nature does blindly, slowly, and ruthlessly, man may do providently, quickly, and kindly." See his 1904 address, *Eugenics: Its Definition, Scope, and Aims.*

in the affirmative. On the other hand, humanity could no longer be seen in terms of a collection of individuals, but rather as an organic whole, as a species, most clearly embodied as the State.[11] These two perspectives had the imprimatur of unassailable science, and citizens in American and Europe began working apace based on those 'facts.'

In *Allowing the Destruction of Life Unworthy of Life*, Hoche argues:

> The mentally dead possess an intellectual level, which we first find at the very bottom of the animal chain, and also the emotions that they feel do not rise above the bar of the most elementary processes, which are associated with animal life.
>
> Therefore, a mentally dead person is also not capable of raising an inner subjective claim to life, just as poorly as he would be capable of other mental processes.
>
> This latter point only appears to be unnecessary; in truth, it has its meaning in the sense that the disposal of a mentally dead person does not equate to any other death. From a purely legal point of view, the destruction of a human life already never means the same.

The distinction between humans and 'animal life' is not drawn very brightly, for Dr. Hoche. Not all deaths are the same. The 'disposal' of a mentally dead person—that is, someone exhibiting an intellect at the level we see among animals—is not the same kind of death as other deaths.

But it is wrong to think only in terms of the individual and his well-being and suffering, according to Hoche. Society itself must endure the burden of these 'useless eaters.' He says:

> Seen from the point of view of a higher civil morality, there is no doubt that exaggerations are being exercised in the striving for the absolute preservation of unworthy life. We have learned, from someone else's point of view, to consider in this respect the state organism as a whole with its own laws and rights, in the same way as, for instance, it would be for a self-contained human or-

---

[11] This is not an assessment about what Darwinism logically entails, but rather a simple recounting of the actual developments according to the record of history.

ganism, which, as us doctors know, surrenders and rejects individual parts or particles that have become worthless or damaged in the interest of the well-being of the whole.

Who is this 'someone' and what is the 'point of view' that Hoche refers to? Whoever this person is, their ideas are a deviation from the "collaboration of the Christian set of ideas" which, according to Hoche, lead to an exaggerated effort to preserve 'life unworthy of life.' He probably does not refer to a particular person's point of view but rather an entirely different framework of understanding, a scientific one, based on Darwinism, that eschews the individual and compels them to look to "the state organism as a whole with its own laws and rights." Just as individual humans jettison "parts or particles that have become worthless or damaged in the interest of the well-being of the whole", the state organism needs to do the same; nay, it is required to, if it is to remain healthy. Death isn't bad. It is actually good, because it strengthens the 'body.'[12]

The import and impact of such notions will vary based on the culture in which it appears. Binding and Hoche were writing shortly after the first world war had ended, with Germany by far the worst for it. The economic conditions that would eventually help spur on public acceptance of the Nazis were probably in view by Hoche, who writes:

> From an economic point of view, these complete retards, just as they meet from very early on all the prerequisites to be classified as fully mentally dead, they would also be at the same time those, whose existence weighs heaviest on society.

He then goes on to calculate the cost required to "care for the retarded" into the billions. That, he says, is just a fraction of the

---

[12] A particular striking example of this perspective can be found in the writings of the German biologist August Weismann, such as this comment in his 1881 essay, *The Duration of Life*. He says: "It is only from the point of view of utility that we can understand the necessity of death" (page 22-23) and on page 24, "Worn-out individuals are not only valueless to the species, but they are even harmful, for they take the place of those which are sound." Weismann invokes natural selection as the mechanism by which the species establishes when an organism will normally die, and makes it clear that this death is good and necessary.

total burden on the state that these people represent, as it does not include all of the private institutions and the 'care personnel' that are 'tied up' by the maintenance "of these empty human shells, some of whom live to be 70 or older."[13]

> The question of whether the necessary expenditure for these categories of cumbersome existence is justified at any cost, was not a pressing one in the past years of prosperity; now things are different, and we must seriously deal with it.

In other words, Germany was ripe to see members of its society as 'ballast' and 'dead-weight.' All of science—in Germany, in England, in the United States—was poised to view humanity in collective, biological, terms, where there was a competition for scarce resources. To their horror, most of those resources were being consumed by inferior elements. But in Germany, following its humiliation in the war, they saw in these scientifically based constructs a way forward:

> Also, with respect to the *scientific* and moral burden on the environment, the mental institution, the state, etc, the feeble-minded are never worth the same.[14]

Hoche said that "the state organism as a whole" had "its own laws and rights." This sentiment was shared by many, both inside of Germany and out.[15] When Hitler and the National Socialists moved to purge Germany of the weak and burdensome *just thirteen years later*, they believed they were acting *scientifically* and with *good* intentions, but according to a "higher civil morality."

This moral plane was beyond the individual, manifesting only at the level of the State, the social organism, and the species.

Hoche believed that *his* was the compassionate view:

> This image will also later show itself in this cultural

---

[13] Margaret Sanger makes a similar argument in her 1922 book, *The Pivot of Civilization*. She rails against 'charity' and all of the money being wasted on the 'unfit.'

[14] Emphasis added.

[15] The reader may wish to consider how different this sentiment is different from contemporary arguments made in the name of the 'common good.' See, for example, arguments for compulsory vaccination.

question of ours. There was a time, which we now view as barbaric, in which the disposal of those born with un-livable conditions was considered natural, and then came the still on-going phase, in which the preservation of any whatsoever worthless existence is ultimately considered the highest moral requirement; there will be a new time, which, from the point of view of a higher morality, will stop to constantly translate into action the demand of a wild humanity concept and an over-protection of the values of existence with heavy sacrifices.

4. Enter: The Experts

From the foregoing, the rough outlines of how Binding and Hoche's book was so well-received in Germany should be clear, but it still doesn't explain how it was that it was a *catalyst*.

Karl Binding and Alfred Hoche were not Nazis. They were not National Socialists. They were academics. Binding was a well-regarded attorney and Hoche was an experienced doctor. *But this is precisely why their views proved instrumental.* It is *because* they were well-respected scholars giving their dispassionate, rational, judgment on whether or not it was ethical to 'dispose' of the 'unworthy' that their arguments had the weight it did. It was because they weren't radical ideologues, but sober academics, that their positions were taken as seriously as they were.

Moreover, *who* took their arguments seriously is critical to observe. It was *the doctors, psychiatrists, and lawyers* that implemented and designed the T4 program and later administrated the extermination camps. It is a myth that these operations were manned by SS thugs pulled out of the German beer halls, willy-nilly. In the words of one survivor of a German concentration camp, the doctors ran it all.[16]

The German 'war on the weak' was viewed by the National Socialists as a medical 'treatment.' Their whole political party was regarded as 'applied biology.'

---

[16] According to the words of one concentration camp prisoner-doctor, as recorded in Robert Jay Clifton's *The Nazi Doctors*, "[Doctors] managed the situation... at the infirmary... selections... at the station... the crematoria... They were everywhere." pg 202.

Hoche, who was married to a Jew and would have one of his own relatives caught up in the Nazi medical dragnet, clearly did not anticipate that *his very own ideas* could be taken in the direction and extent that they ended up going. This is certainly the case with Binding, who died in 1920. In this book, both put some considerable emphasis on the 'consenting' and 'voluntary' nature of the ideas they were proposing.[17] This philosophical distinction did not prove to be a very high hurdle for the Nazis on their way to exercising "the state organism's [...] own laws and rights."

You should hear what the scholars, doctors, and academics are saying today! On their view, they are just having 'a conversation.' So too were Binding and Hoche, who no doubt would have been annoyed with the fact that their book would become linked with the Holocaust. Savulescu, likewise, chafes at the outrage inspired by his ideas or the forum he gives to similar ones.

For example, two of his friends in academia, Alberto Giubilini and Francesca Minerva, published an article titled "After-birth abortion: why should the baby live" in Savulescu's bioethics journal. Their argument was that a born child is not fundamentally different than an unborn child, so if we accept aborting an unborn child, we should not have any objection to aborting *born* children. This is offensive to many... but they are correct. Based on their notions of what people really are (just another kind of animal) and in what sense people have value (only insofar as society or the state assigns it), *they are correct.* So, if *you* accept those premises yourself but find yourself repulsed by their viewpoint, *you* have a problem. *You* are not being consistent. *They* are.

Giubilini and Minerva continue:

Nonetheless, to bring up such children[18] might be an unbearable burden on the family and on society as a whole, when the state economically provides for their

---

[17] Binding more explicitly than Hoche, but realize that Hoche felt that the mentally retarded were on the level of the animals, for whom no 'consent' was possible, and therefore not really relevant.

[18] Disabled children, such as children with Down Syndrome.

care.

Here, in a publication from 2012, is a concise restatement of Binding and Hoche's own arguments and approach. It is but a very small step from this to a state acting according to its own interests based on 'laws and rights' that manifest at the level of the state—setting aside the interests of the parents completely. The only difference with the Nazis is that they made that step in logic, and had the power to act on it.

Giubilini and Minerva don't take that step, but 'bioethicist' Jacob Appel comes as close to the edge as you can without going over it, arguing that only doctors and state officials have the objectivity required to do the 'compassionate' thing and end a 'life unworthy of life.'[19] Appel says that such 'neonatal euthanasia' is the "inevitable consequence of our progress toward liberal humanism."[20]

Savulescu came to Giubilini and Minerva's defense saying,

> As Editor of the Journal, I would like to defend its publication. The arguments presented, in fact, are largely not new and have been presented repeatedly in the academic literature and public fora by the most eminent philosophers and bioethicists in the world, including Peter Singer, Michael Tooley and John Harris in defence of infanticide, which the authors call after-birth abortion. [...]
> The authors provocatively argue that there is no moral difference between a fetus and a newborn. Their capacities are relevantly similar. If abortion is permissible, infanticide should be permissible. *The authors proceed logically from premises which many people accept to a conclusion that many of those people would reject.* [...]
> What is disturbing is not the arguments in this paper nor its publication in an ethics journal. It is the hostile, abusive, threatening responses that it has elicited. More than ever, *proper academic discussion and freedom* are under threat from fanatics opposed to *the very values of*

---

[19] My characterization; Appel of course doesn't use the phrase, but the meaning is more or less the same.

[20] Jacob Appel, Neonatal Euthanasia: Why Require Parental Consent? Bioethical Inquiry (2009).

a liberal society. [emphasis added]

You see, says Savulescu, these ideas are not new! Singer, Tooley, Harris... and, we may mention, Binding and Hoche... have all made them as well. These scholars are not advocating for these views, rather, they are merely providing sober conclusions from the facts. The ideas merely "proceed from premises which many people accept." They are not radical ideologues. They are well-respected academics merely participating in "the very values of a liberal society."

What could possibly go wrong?

Savulescu, Giubilini, Minerva, and Appel do not imagine that their arguments and positions could possibly lead to any kind of atrocity a decade hence. For them, ideas are toys. They are playthings for intellectuals. They are not men and women of action. But men and women of action are everywhere. Like the scholars, these men and women of action believe they are good people. In fact, we will assume they are. Our men and women of action do not see themselves as 'bioethicists.' Most consider these issues 'above their pay grade.' They are relying on people like Savulescu, etc, to find answers to these difficult questions for them, and are thankful for their efforts. Likewise, the scientists and medical professionals in Germany throughout the 1920s were thankful that Binding and Hoche did the heavy lifting for them. And why not? *That's why we have experts.*

We are pinning an awful lot on Binding and Hoche, but in truth they were just two very prominent examples within the worldwide scholarly community. They would surely protest as Savelecsu did, pointing out that that their argumets were "largely not new and have been presented repeatedly ... by the most eminent philosophers and bioethicists..." They woud have differed only in the list of names they would have then added.

Thus we must recognize that it was an unquestioning deference to experts that played a large part in turning the academic musings of *Allowing the Destruction of Life Unworthy of Life* into one of history's worst nightmares. Binding and Hoche merely crystallized what was already being argued by experts around the world.

Both the common man and the uncommon politician feel that it is quite reasonable to act in accordance to the recommendations by those with expertise. Certainly, we must make an allowance for the valuable contributions that experts can make, but their position of prestige is particular manifestation of power, just as much as political office is. As such, it needs to be subjected to checks and balances just as any other power is. The most obvious and easiest 'check and balance' is to critically evaluate, test, and challenge whatever it is the experts place in front of you for consideration.

The vast majority of people in the 1920s and 1930s, not just in Germany, but everywhere, simply assumed that the scholars and doctors could be trusted. If they said something was true and for the 'common good' it probably was. In hindsight, we can think of a thousand ways that these people were wrong. If we will learn from the past, we must catch our errors *before* they turn horrific—not in hindsight. That means we must challenge experts the way we challenge any who are influential.

5. Thou Shalt Not Suffer

Finally, we must call attention to the *utilitarian* philosophy that is seen in Binding and Hoche's work.

Evolutionary theory is supposed to account for every aspect of the human being. Through natural selection, our brains and bodies and so on and so forth have changed over time resulting finally in the human species. If one jettisons God from this analysis—and most evolutionists believe one should—then even our moral behavior is the result of unguided (by definition!) selective processes over time.

'Morality' is an artifact, the result of physical processes as much as our ear lobes are. Darwin showed that morality was something that could, and should, be understood in biological terms. 'Survival of the fittest' was not seen as only an astute observation by Darwin, but a moral mandate.

However, many people were not comfortable leaving it only at that. Darwin himself argued that we should see our humanitarian sympathies as somehow a result of natural selection, since, after all, we do have humanitarian views, and they must have come from *somewhere*.

With God no longer a viable candidate for reasonable people, the search was on for an ethical system based on objective science that was consistent with Darwinism. John Stuart Mill was once again advancing utilitarianism just as Darwin's theory was gaining currency.[21]

In its broad outlines, utilitarianism holds that the 'right' choice is the one that produces the most good, for the most people. This 'good' can often be measured, and isn't something scientific if it is objective and can be measured?

But there are three obvious problems.

First of all, how are we to define 'good'? Second of all, doesn't invoking the 'most good for the most people' necessarily imply that there will be some people who will not be able to partake of the 'most good'? Thirdly, *who* decides?

To the first, the answer given by utilitarians from Jeremy Bentham to Mill to Peter Singer[22] is that 'good' is more or less that which brings happiness, and thus conversely, 'bad' is more or less what results in suffering. Happiness, then, is the highest good, and suffering becomes the worst evil.

This emphasis on suffering is succintly expressed by Bentham:

> ...a full-grown horse or dog, is beyond comparison a more rational, as well as a more conversable animal, than an infant of a day or a week or even a month, old. But suppose the case were otherwise, what would it avail? The question is not, Can they *reason*? nor, Can they *talk*? but, Can they *suffer*?

Unfortunately, it is not practically possible to make everyone happy at the same time. Thus, calculations that involve weighing the happiness of some against the suffering of others is inevitable. The easiest way to make such calculations is to put dollar values on people. As you will see, Binding and Hoche felt that they were equipped to make such calculations, but history shows that this task did not in fact fall to them. Who decided? The Nazis.

Far from being an out-dated and discarded ethical system, utilitarian analysis is pervasive in contemporary society. It con-

---

[21] Indeed, Darwin and Mill were friends. Darwin refers to Mill's writings in some of his own works.

[22] Mentioned earlier by Savulescu in his defense of Giubilini and Minerva.

tinues to appeal to people because of its apparent neutrality and the intuition that we should prefer happiness over suffering. However, it still tends to operate by assigning monetary values to human lives, most easily recognized today in health care rationing, but manifesting in numerous contexts. The growing movement to legalize physician-assisted suicide and euthanasia also has a strong utilitarian streak to it. Abortion and infanticide (in particular, in cases of birth defects) are justified on the same grounds.[23]

These arguments are in many cases virtually indistinguishable from Binding and Hoche's. Now, like then, the presumption is that these life and death calculations will be made by individuals, parents, and maybe doctors. However, there is no logical reason why the State should not be prepared to step in and make such decisions, especially when the individuals, parents, and doctors won't make the right ones.

Besides, doesn't the State have a unique obligation to administer the nation's resources wisely, fairly, and justly? The individual need concern himself only with his own life, health, and resources. The State, in its great benevolence, must think of everyone, and, as such, follow a slightly different and distinctly higher set of laws and principles.

What could go wrong?

---

[23] See for example *Practical Ethics*, a textbook written by prominent utilitarian Peter Singer, who writes in chapter 7, 'Taking Life: Humans': "In dealing with an objection to the view of abortion presented in Chapter 6, we have already looked beyond abortion to infanticide. In so doing, we will have confirmed the suspicion of supporters of the sanctity of human life that once abortion is accepted, euthanasia lurks around the corner—and for them, euthanasia is an unequivocal evil." Singer objects: "...it is the refusal to accept killing that, in some cases, is horrific." Page 175 in the second edition.

6. Summary

Let us see if we can sum up some of the right lessons[24] to draw from the horrors of the 20th century.[25]

1. Deference to 'experts,' including deference by 'experts' to other 'experts,' *is dangerous*. Any such deference must be thoughtful and deliberative and not automatic. The power and authority of 'experts' must be subject to checks and balances like any other power and authority.

2. Allowing ethical considerations regarding life and death to be linked to the interests of the 'social organism' *is dangerous*.

3. Believing that there is one set of moral principles for the 'individual' and another set for the 'social organism' *is dangerous*.

4. You cannot get an 'ought' from an 'is.' Asserting that certain ethical considerations, behaviors, and attitudes flow directly from scientific data *is dangerous*.

5. Behaving as though ideas—even grotesque, inhuman, ideas—can be carefully considered for their relative merits as though they have no consequences or implications *is dangerous*.

6. Utilitarianism, especially when applied to a large group of people simultaneously by a small group of people (experts, usually), *is dangerous*.

Now, in calling these things 'dangerous,' the purpose is not to dismiss any of them out of hand. Remember, we are leaving open the possibility that one really could have a conversation about, say, for example, killing born children just because they have a disability, without anyone actually trying to implement it in the real world—ever. What happened with Binding and Hoche's work is that their ideas found an audience in a particular culture that was uniquely primed to embrace *and* implement them. Can we be so certain that ten years from now there will not be another similar society?

Does it matter that our own culture has embraced these atti-

---

[24] Where 'right' means, "that which can help us prevent such horrors.'

[25] I hope by now it is realized that the Holocaust is not by any means the only atrocity referred to and Nazism the only place where the ideas under examination were, and are, held.

tudes but our governments lack the 'free hand' that the National Socialists had in implementing them? That is, if these ideas are pervasive even now, does the fact that some modern democracies presently serve as a check against abuses provide any comfort, especially as various governments, including the United States federal government, move to insulate themselves against those checks and balances?[26]

These questions are left for your consideration. The worst thing you could do is ignore them, for failing to learn the lessons of history, while not necessarily destining you to repeat them, certainly opens up the very real possibility that you could make them again, *without even knowing you are doing it.*

7. Conclusion

Battle lines have developed around the horrors of the 20th century. Weinberg, you will recall, said it takes *religion* to make good people do evil things. To that end, there is a great effort to pin the Hitler and the Holocaust on *Christians*, and in the spirit of 'ideas have consequences', secular humanists have tried to argue that really, really, really bad things will happen if religious people are able to express their religious views within the public sphere—the Holocaust a case in point.

Certainly, there are ways in which the Nazis can be shown to have embraced things we might properly call 'religious.' These things, in the main, were *pagan*, not Christian. They were chosen because they were consistent with the Nazi's 'scientific racism.'

This matter cannot be settled here, but as you will soon see, Binding and Hoche perceived that Christianity was an obstacle in the way of the really compassionate program of ending 'lives unworthy of life.'

Binding specifically says "that religious reasons hold no evidential value in the eyes of the Law." He adds, "the Law is secular through and through." He clearly supports the notion that in secular affairs there must be a strict 'separation of church and

---

[26] For example, in Britain, with the Liverpool Care Pathway, or in the United States with the coming implementation of the Independent Payment Advisory Board, which will have the power to decide who gets what care, based on the standards that it alone is able to set and consider.

state.'[27]

Both Binding and Hoche exhibit contempt for Christianity's historic defense of 'lives unworthy of life.' Binding regards the Church's opposition to a 'right to suicide' as unchristian. He is pleased to report that this right has been "fully re-won [...] apart from very few less *evolved* countries." [emphasis added.] Hoche regards the time "in which the preservation of any whatsoever worthless existence is ultimately considered the highest moral requirement" as barbaric.

Binding says, and repeats: "I can find absolutely no reason, from a legal, social, moral, religious point of view, not to allow those that want it, to kill those beyond salvation, who desperately desire it."

Both Binding and Hoche believed that their even-handed approach to the issue had nothing whatsoever to do with religious beliefs. What Christians in the past had regarded as barbaric, Binding and Hoche endorse. What Binding and Hoche regard as barbaric, the Church embraced.

The Nazis sided with Binding and Hoche with a wholly unanticipated enthusiasm. While there may have been 'religious' components to the Third Reich, their killing programs were seen by them as part of their *secular* efforts.

Dr. Anthony Horvath

Director of the Policy Intersections Research Center

www.policyintersections.com

---

[27] Hitler takes a very similar view, saying, "I know that here and there the objection has been raised: Yes, but you have deserted Christianity. No, it is not that we have deserted Christianity; it is those who came before us who deserted Christianity. We have only carried through a clear division between politics, which have to do with terrestrial things, and religion, which must concern itself with the celestial sphere. There has been no interference with the doctrine of the Confessions or with their religious freedom, nor will there be any such interference. On the contrary the State protects religion, though always on the one condition that religion will not be used as a cover for political ends."

Further Reading:

For an extensive look at the role of doctors in ushering in the Holocaust, read *The Nazi Doctors: Medical Killing and the Psychology of Genocide by Robert Jay Lifton*. Part I of this book is entitled "Life Unworthy of Life: 'The Genetic Cure.'" Nearly a hundred pages of this book is dedicated to exploring the progression from academic musings through the extermination of 'lives unworthy of lives' in the T4 program on the way to the full-blown Holocaust.

For an extensive look at the role acceptance of Darwinism had in the development of Nazi ideology, read *From Darwin to Hitler: Evolutionary Ethics, Eugenics, and Racism in Germany* by Richard Weikart. Weikart explicitly denies that evolutionary theory *necessarily* leads to Nazism, but shows conclusively that the Nazis thought they were acting on the basis of Darwinian science.

For an exposition on how Binding and Hoche's ideas are accepted and implemented today, read Wesley J. Smith's *Culture of Death: The Assault on Medical Ethics in America*. An entire chapter entitled "Life Unworthy of Life" puts Binding and Hoche's book into broader context and gives numerous modern day examples of the same ideas in action.

Another book that has an entire chapter titled "Life Unworthy of Life" is Gene Edward Veith's *Modern Fascism: Liquidating the Judeo-Christian Worldview*. This one comes with a twist, showing that Nazism wasn't the only '-ism' that embraced Binding and Hoche's conclusions. More than the other books in this list, Veith's endeavors to show how these other '-isms' saw themselves in conflict with a Christian worldview.

Other works that may be useful include Daniel J. Kevles' *In the Name of Eugenics* and Edwin Black's *War on the Weak*. Both document the close relationships between eugenicists in Germany and in the United States and warn of a coming 'Newgenics.'

ALLOWING THE DESTRUCTION OF LIFE UNWORTHY OF LIFE.

ITS MEASURE AND FORM.

by

Jurist and Law Professor Karl Binding, PhD.
University of Leipzig.

Doctor and Medical Professor Alfred Hoche, M.D.
University of Freiburg.

Karl Binding ✝

Privy councilor Binding was called upon during
the preparation of this manuscript; the response
that followed is from the voice of the dead.

I dare say, that the questions that we deal with in
this paper are the after-thoughts on the subject of
the deceased that originated from the most vivid
sense of responsibility and the deepest love of
mankind.

Personally, I will always recollect with nostalgia
the hour of the common work with the hot-head
full of cool understanding.

Freiburg, Switzerland, April 10, 1920.

Hoche.

I.

Legal Arguments

by
Jurist and Law
Professor Karl Binding, PhD.

At the end of my life, I dare raise another question that has occupied my mind for several years, and which has however been timidly passed on by most, because it is considered a delicate question with a difficult solution; making sure that this question is not phrased wrongly is a matter here of "an inflexible point in our moral and social perception."

Here it goes: should the lawful destruction of life, as per today's laws–prompted by a desperate situation -, be limited to suicide, or should it be legally extended to include the killing of others, and under which circumstances?

Dealing with this question takes us from case group to case group, whose situation shakes us all most deeply. It is extremely important not to leave the final word on this matter to emotions of excessive concern, but rather leave it to deliberate legal consideration of the reasons for and the arguments against the approval of this question. Only on such solid foundations will it be possible to build anything further.

I therefore put the heaviest weight on a strict juridical handling [of this question]. Consequently, the solid starting point for us can only be found in the current laws: to what extent is–again under desperate circumstances–the killing of a human life really *allowed* today, and what are we supposed to understand from that? The concept of "allowing" it leads to the recognition of killing rights.

These [rights] remain here fully ignored.

The scientific clarification of the pertinent starting point is however so essential, since the latter is interpreted very often either wrongly or very imprecisely.

I. Today's Legal Nature of Suicide.
The So-Called Complicity in It.

I. From a power, which he cannot oppose, man is lifted into existence for man. To find himself with such a fate– this is his life property. He is the only one that can determine what to do with it within the tight confines of his freedom of movement. In this respect, he is the born ruler over his own life.

The law–helpless to let the individual determine how much of the load that life thrusts upon him he is able to carry–finds its extreme expression of this concept in the recognition of everyone's freedom to end his own life. After long, highly unchristian undermining of this recognition– demanded by the Church, supported by the impure view that a God of Love could want man to die only after endless agony of the body and soul, - today [this recognition] has been fully re-won–apart from very few less evolved countries–and should remain an unchallenged right for all future to come.

This freedom should have been the first of all "human rights" under Natural Law.

II. It is however by far still not clear how this freedom should be viewed in the realm of our political rights. This uncertainty can be seen just as well through the wrong terminology, as the wrong practical conclusions. It is just about time that better scientific accuracy solved the, as of yet, unclear treatment of these questions - in particular, that

2

the fundamental legal difference between the badly so-called suicide and the killing of a consenting person be clearly recognized.

There are currently two totally contradicting parallel opinions regarding suicide–both unanimous only in the fact that they are both wrong and that they both stand upon the postulate of their impunity.

I. According to the former view, suicide is an illegal action, a crime, most closely related to murder and manslaughter, because it violates the ban on killing a person.

Such extension of the rule on killing is very foreign to our normal system, and it lacks any proof for the criminal nature of suicide. All religious reasons hold no evidential value in the eyes of the Law for two reasons. They rely here completely on an unworthy understanding of God, and the Law is secular through and through: based on the rules of public community life. Incidentally, the new testament has no word on the subject.

Incidentally, the same elementary power that proves the illegality of suicide,[28] applies equally well to the unfounded "pharisaic" (Gaupp) claim that [suicide] is always an immoral action and therefore its illegality is self-evident.

The "harsh and loveless" term 'suicide' itself is biased. Because the "murder"[29] always required cowardly secret and despicable acts. And now take into consideration the large number of mentally disturbed people that hurt themselves! In addition, there are selfless suicides of people of sound mind, with the highest morals, while on the other

---

[28] The term "suicide" is derived from the two Latin words "sew" (of oneself) and "cidium" (a killing or slaying). The German term, as used in the original manuscript ("Selbstmord"), is closer to the original meaning of the word than the English term, so that the meaning in German is self-evident in the word itself, and the author can therefore use it as a play of words to make his point across. The literal translation of the German term would be "self-murder" (*TN*)

[29] Referring again to the German word for suicide, which is literally translated as "self-murder" (*TN*)

hand, there are also suicides that can sink down to the lowest level of frivolous meanness or awful cowardice. Yes, there are failed suicides, which earn stern moral reprimand just because of the failure.

Aside from that, the moral conduct as such is also not necessarily illegal, and the legal conduct not always necessarily moral.

The evidence of the unlawfulness of suicide can only be found through the exact proof of the pertinent rule on killing. The material for this task is however completely missing, since suicide is neither classified as punishable nor otherwise unequivocally defined as a crime. Alternatively, [the evidence] could be reached as a conclusion from established legal premises. Feuerbach tried [to get] such proof, but in the most inadequate way. " Whoever enters the state–the newborn does not enter!–obliges his virtues to the state and acts unlawfully when he arbitrarily robs the state of them through suicide". This is an obvious meaningless *petitio principii*.

Therefore, not only is all supporting evidence for the criminal nature of suicide missing, but, these days, no suicide victim or anyone else administering it would ever in the slightest think of viewing suicide as a forbidden action and to really place it qualitatively on the same scale as murder and manslaughter.

Those, however, who support the crime view, must consider the so-called accomplice in the suicide as a criminal under any circumstance. And with regards to the impunity of suicide, that of the "accomplice" deserves by no means any further consideration: since they take illegal action on the life of a third party, therefore, this action stands on a higher level of punishment than that of those who abuse only themselves, if that act is viewed as a crime.

As a consequence of the view of the criminal nature of suicide, the state organs that deal with preventing crime have a necessary duty to prevent the death of the suicidal person and his so-called accomplice, against which the latter have obviously no self-defense right.

The opposite view stems from the Natural Law's point of view, even though not always completely supported by the Natural Law teachings, which are heavily influenced by the Church view: suicide is the exercise of one's killing right. This position also has no supporting evidence, since the impunity of suicide, i.e. its immunity from punishment, cannot be derived simply from its lack of punishment. There are plenty of unpunished crimes.

Therefore this is a purely theoretical construction, which is guilty of a complete misjudgment of the nature of subjective rights and of the usual confusion of the reflex effect of prohibiting such rights. Since only the killing of another human being is prohibited, it must be concluded that every man has a right either to life, in life or even over life–all three views are equally used -, and by virtue of this possession right, he is allowed to incidentally claim that this life is fighting against him, and he has therefore the killing right to himself or against himself, he may even be able to bestow this [right] onto others on his behalf.

If I base the impossible right to or in or over one's own life on itself for once–very nicely in contrast to E. Rupp (Pg. 8)–it is then necessary to object to the notion of the right to commit suicide, since rights on actions are awarded only for purposes that are generally viewed as conforming and useful to the legal system. This notion therefore contains a general approval of the action, which is granted as a right. This is however absolutely impossible for suicide. In a large number of instances, however, this [action] has very sensitive harmful effects on the legal sphere: like grounds for more extensive public support obligations. It can indeed become the means for infringement on more serious legal duties: like the duties, not to pay any school tuition, not to serve any punishment, to serve as outpost for the enemy in dangerous situations, or take part in an attack.

If however we stand from the viewpoint of the recognition of the legality of suicide, then it can be concluded a.) that no one can have a right to hinder the suicidal person in their legal act;

b) that the latter has a right to self-defense against any interference attempt;

c) that, if we consider the right of a human being to end their life as a transferable right, all so-called accomplices that act with his noted consent–but absolutely only these–act just as legally, and can therefore not be hindered by anyone and can act in self-defense against any such interference attempt.

However, any accomplices that act without such consent, taking part in *re illicita*, may, must eventually be stopped from carrying out their actions, and make themselves basically guilty of the crime, if successful.

Yes, from the starting point of this transferable killing right, it even follows that

d) the killing of the noted consenting victim must be viewed as a legal killing act.

III. If suicide can neither be considered a criminal nor a lawful act, then the only thing that remains is to view it as a legally unbannable action. This notion, which freely appears more and more frequently in various legal formulations, is rooted in a different reason, whose difference can in this case be based on itself. I have previously voiced my opinion on the matter as follows: the law, as the order of human community life, "is reluctant to transfer the divorce between legal subject and legal object to the individual and to make the latter the author of this dualism, based on which he must accept also for himself quality goods, or maybe event things, so that he can obtain legal rights and legal responsibilities for himself."

Nothing else remains then for the law, but to consider a living human being as the ruler over his existence and over the form of his existence. As a result of this, there are very important consequences:

1. This recognition is true only for the life's owner himself. Only his actions against himself cannot be prohi-

bited.

2. This recognition does not provide any exception to the killing ban; since the latter only deals with the killing of others, consequently suicide, [i.e. the killing of oneself], is not prohibited.

3. All so-called complicity in the suicide falls under the rule on killing, is therefore illegal, and can, must, be punished under the circumstances, otherwise, if that is not possible, he is not to blame. "Can" here refers to: *de lege ferenda*, "must" refers to: *de lege lata*, in the event that the so-called accomplice shares in or originates the act.

4. Only the action of the deceased cannot be prohibited. Through his consent, he is completely powerless to make the actions of others unbannable as well. For good reason, our positive law views the killing of the consenting victim as a crime.

5. If the action cannot be prohibited for him, then nobody can hinder him, if he is capable enough to understand what he is doing; he then has a right to self-defense against any interference; trying to force him to desist from his actions is illegal coercion.

These suicide rescuers act mostly in *optima fide* and then go unpunished. A strong case in support for their standpoint is made by the experience that the rescued suicide victim is often very happy about his rescue and, in most cases, forgoes a second attempt after the first one failed.

IV. The legal and social weak point of allowing all suicides is the loss of the large number of still very vital lives, whose carriers are simply too lazy or coward to carry on any further with what life has bestowed upon them.

This [point] weighs heavy on the scale for the assessment of the guilt of the so-called accomplice. The conscious assisted suicide of the terminally ill weighs significantly less than that of the healthy, who wants to evade his creditors.

II. The Pure Case of Euthanasia

With the Proper Boundaries Does Not Require Any Special Approval.

It would appear, and as far as a purely causal consideration is concerned, without any doubt, that the killing of a third party, which forms the basis for the so-called euthanasia, is, to my knowledge, still not being punished under the law, as of yet.

I. The ugly name of "assisted death", which has surfaced in the new literature, is ambiguous. Here, the painkilling means, which do not affect the cause of death from the illness, must not be taken into any consideration at all. Only the displacement of a painful, maybe even longer-lasting, cause of death, which is rooted in the illness, with a less painful alternative is of significance for our considerations. The doctor, or maybe another assistant, gives a deadly morphine injection, which is painless, possibly quicker, but maybe also a little slower at bringing death, to a lung cancer patient in terrible pain.

II. Regarding the legal nature of this action, its unlawfulness or its unbanning–since it is impossible to speak of a subjective right of its execution–rises the same, in my opinion totally unnecessary, argument as over the nature of the doctor's–more correctly of the one aiming to heal–apparent interference in the health, and especially in the bodily integrity, of another.

The situation, in which this action of euthanasia is planned, must however be very clearly specified: the internally ill or wounded, who faces death from his illness or wound, which also brings him pain, as a matter of fact already now and before, so that the time difference between death from the illness and that through external means does not come into consideration. Then, it is absolutely not possible to speak of a considerable shortening of the life time of the dying, or at best only a narrow pedant would be able to do so.

Therefore, if somebody gives the deadly morphine injection to a paralytic, at their request or maybe even without it, at the beginning of their condition, which may well continue for years–in this case it is not possible to speak of a pure case of euthanasia. Here a strong shortening of the life, which also makes a difference in the eyes of the law, has taken place, which is not permissible without legal approval.

III. At the same time, it is however clear that: the sure cause of an agonizing death was definitively established, the imminent death was in clear sight. Nothing has been changed in this threatening death situation, except the exchange of this existing cause of death with another of equal effect, which is however painless. This is no "Act of killing in the legal sense", but rather only an adaptation of the already irrevocable cause of death, which can no longer be prevented: it is in reality a pure healing act. "The removal of pain is also an act of healing."

Such behavior could only be viewed as prohibited killing if the law system were barbaric enough to allow that the terminally ill should definitely die through their agonies. Today, this is no longer acceptable.

It is shameful that anybody could have ever thought of this, even acted this way!

IV. Therefore, it can be concluded that: this is by no means the case of a statutory exception to the ruling on killing, of an illegal killing, in case it was not possible to expressly recognize an exception from this, but rather it is a matter of unbannable healing work of blessed effect for deeply agonizing sick people, of a shortening of the suffering for those that are still living, as long as they are still alive, and not in truth about their killing.

Therefore, this action must be viewed as unbannable, even when the law does not even mention its recognition.

And, truthfully, there is actually no real need for the consent of the suffering patient. Obviously the action cannot be taken against their prohibition, but in many many cases the subjects of this healing intervention are momentarily unconscious. From the nature of this action, it also results that assistance to this action and the provision for a third party are equally unprohibitive. The erroneous assumption of the deathly situation that leads to an act of euthanasia can make the person guilty of involuntary manslaughter.

III. Signs For Additional Concessions.

Our initial examination provided the following results: today, suicide is absolutely the only form of killing that cannot be prohibited under any circumstance. At the moment, allowing its so-called complicity is completely out of the question. This is because the latter is of a criminal nature in all its forms. It cannot be absolved of its criminal nature even through the consent of the suicide victim. However, after execution of the accessory action of the so-called complicity, the Civil Code's position will be that assistance to the suicide should remain unpunished and that it may find its incitement to the act in the deliberate regulation of suicide according to Regulation § 48 of the German Civil Code—no matter whether the suicide victim is competent or not.

A further concession could therefore only be allowing the killing of another. This would actually accomplish what allowing suicide does not: an actual restriction of the legal outlawing of killing.

Something different has recently been entered for such [an action], and the expression of "the right to die" was coined as the keyword for this action .

This does not really cover an actual right over death, but it rather simply describes a recognized claim for certain people to be relieved from an unbearable life.

This new direction is paved through two tendencies, of

which the former, the more radical one, was formed in the *a priori* field of legal interpreted theory, while the latter, more careful and cautious, was based on the legislation.

I. It is known, that the Romans let the killing of the consenting victim go unpunished. Based on a completely exaggerated interpretation of the I. 1 § 5 D *de injuriis* 47, 10: *quia nulla injuria est, quae in voentem fit*, which simply refers to the Roman private crime of *injuria*, the natural rights doctrine was completely redone based on the enormous power of consent by the injured towards the injury. This excluded, without exception, the illegality of the injury whenever the consequence of this consent could be recognized in any way, as long as there was anyone at all injured in the crime: the action could therefore not be punished at all, since any injury suffered willingly by the victim, especially his killing, was a non-prohibitive action.

This position was used in the last century by W. v. Humboldt (Collective Works, vol. VII p. 138), Henke and Wächter, and later especially by Ortmann, Rödenbeck, Keßler, Klee, and E. Rupp. If they were to remain consistent, they would have surely become strong opponents of the German Civil Code. § 216.

II. The passing within the legislation relates equally to the consent in the injury, which was elevated to the desire to be injured in the interest of a clearer recognition and easier provability.

This killing request becomes a reason for mitigation of punishment, the killing from a request therefore still remains a true crime–a crime of course not in the sense of the Penal Code. § 1.

This is how the Prussian Common Law Part II Section 20 § 834 started. Several German Penal Codes followed, but not yet the Bavarian version of 1813; rather first [was] the Saxon version of 1838. Also the Prussian one reacted negatively [on the subject matter], just like its successors, the one from Oldenburg in 1858 and the Bavarian one from 1861, but not the Lübeck (f. § 145) one.

This dismissal of the desire as a reason for a mitigation of punishment compelled a terribly harsh conclusion, namely to assign the punishment of murder or manslaughter to the consented killing.

This unendurable necessity also led, in the third drafting of the Northern German Penal Code–the first two were really silent on the matter! - to the incorporation of the killing, where the death had been expressly and truly desired, to "pass" as independent killing and therefore to fall under the still too high prison punishment of no less than 3 years. This proposal later found its way unchanged in the legislation. It is subject to the correct understanding of a necessary recognizable reason for mitigation of punishment.

[By default], the killing of the consenting victim does not need to break the will to live of the victim, which is the cause of what leads to the terrible severity [of the punishment] awarded for the regular killing.

Here lies the reason for initially considering the criminal meaning of killing the consenting victim as objectively less important. On the subjective side, this goes hand in hand with a mitigation of the blame, when the action was driven by compassion. This is however not at all necessary for the mitigation of punishment–neither from a theoretical point of view, nor from *de lege lata*. However, the consent to the killing, which has been elevated to a desire [to be killed], does not lead to a mitigation of punishment under *de lege lata*.

The legal weak points of this privileged form of deliberate killing are three: 1. the legal elevation of the consent to a desire, or even to the expressed desire, forces [us] to handle the killing of those that are not included in this higher form of consent as murder or common manslaughter;

2. the law does not distinguish between the destruction of worthy and worthless life;

3. the law does a favor also to the very cruel killings. The latter of these flaws has however been clearly recognized by a number of our penal codes.

Five of our penal codes, first among which the Württemberg version of 1839 (U. 239), recognize a double privileged killing crime: namely, the killing from the [victim's] desire performed to a "terminally ill or mortally wounded" person.

Here we clearly see the idea emerge, that such a life no longer deserves the fullest punishment protection, and that the desire to its destruction should receive a greater legal consideration than the desire to destroy a vital life.

However, this very good start did not find any continuation in the German Criminal Law, but in contrast found a very lively reception in the literature!

IV. Should the Grounds Which Mitigate Killing Offenses Become Grounds for Allowing the Killing of a Third Party?

Considering that a whole number of famous jurists completely overturn the illegality of the consent in the killing, so that the killing of the consenting victim can always be handled as unprohibitive, and that, on the other hand, in recent years, voices strongly moved and filled with noble compassion for people suffering unbearably are being raised so loud in favor of allowing the killing of such suffering people, it is therefore natural to say: there is therefore at the moment still the question in terms of *de lege ferenda*, of whether maybe one or the other of these reasons for mitigation of punishment could be elevated to a legal reason for an exemption from punishment or whether at least, if both are met, there are grounds for privileges: if consent and unbearable suffering make the killing justified, does this mean that the latter should be viewed as unprohibitive?

It is not of no interest to see that the authors of the preliminary draft of 1909 absolutely rejected the privileges of those, "who, out of compassion, rob the life of the hopelessly ill without their request".

How behind [with the times] are these present lawmakers compared to the Prussian Land Law, whose Part II Lit. XX § 833 stated in such a magnanimous way for those days, and at the same time so exquisite from a legal point of view that: "Those who shorten the life of the mortally wounded or otherwise terminally ill, supposedly with good intentions, should be considered equal to committing involuntary manslaughter according to § 778.779." The threatened punishment is very mild: prison or house arrest "from one month up to two years".

Over one hundred years have passed on the land, and such costly statutes have brought no rewards to the German people!

The Norwegian Penal Code of May 22nd, 1902 § 235 gives the same rights of punishable offense for such a killing as for the killing of the consenting victim. The motive for the German draft from 1909 is explained as follows: such provision could "be misused in worse ways and put the life of sick people in considerable danger", and it is also practically impossible to find suitable wording for it.

I. I would like now to separate both threads for just a moment, to tie them back together again later, so as to put forth the preliminary issue once and for all, which, in my opinion, must now absolutely be said. The legal, apparently so businesslike formulation, sounds very heartless: in truth, it stems only from the deepest compassion.

Are there any human lives, which have so strongly lost the quality of being the object of legal protection, that their continuation both for the person in question and the society has permanently lost any value?"

It is sufficient to just pose this question and an uneasy feeling stirs in anybody that has become used to treasure the value of the single life for the individual and for the community. He reckons with pain, how wasteful we are with the most valuable life, filled with the largest will to live and the biggest vitality, and the life that gets away from him, and what measure of often totally useless wasted labor, patience and financial expenditure we spend on it to keep a worthless life for so long, until nature–often so uncompassionately late–robs it of the last chance of continuation.

Consider at the same time a battlefield constantly covered with dead youth, or a mine, where methane gas has buried hundreds of diligent workers, and compare this to our mental institute with its care for its living residents–and one is deeply shaken by this glaring discord between the sacrifice of the most expensive goodness of humanity on the largest scale on one hand, and the greatest care, not only totally worthless but rather going against valuable existence, on the other side.

There is by no means any doubt that there are living people, whose death is a relief for them and at the same time it frees the society and especially the state from a burden, whose life, aside from being an example of greater selflessness, does not offer the smallest use.

Is it however really like that–is there indeed human life, to which further holding onto has permanently lost any reasonable interest–then the legal system is faced with the fatal question of whether it has the duty, in active practice for their social continuation–especially also through the full use of the protection from punishment–to intervene or to allow its destruction under specific conditions? It is also possible to pose the question from a legislative point of view there: whether the energetic retention of such a life earns at all the merit as proof for the unassailability of life, or whether allowing the termination of such a life, which is liberating for all people involved, appears to be the lesser evil?

II. Hardly any doubt can prevail after cool calculated logic about the necessity to provide an answer. I strongly believe, however, that a definitive answer should not be given exclusively through calculated reasoning: its content must receive approval through the deep feeling of its correctness. Each unprohibitive killing of a third party must be perceived at the very least as a relief by that person: otherwise, its permission is forbidden by itself. This, however, leads to an absolutely necessary follow-up: the full attention to the will to live of all people, even the sickest and the most suffering and the most useless ones.

The legal system can never allow going ahead with the actions of those killers and manslaughterers, who have forcefully broken their victim's will to live.

Also the issue of allowing the killing of the most feeble-minded, who feel good about their life, is obviously out of the question.

III. The people that come under consideration now fall, as far as I can see, into two large groups, between which it is possible to find a middle one.

1. those [people that are] lost because of an illness or wound, which is beyond salvation, and who, with a full understanding of their condition, have the urgent wish to be liberated and have somehow made this known.

Here, both previously mentioned grounds for privileges are met. I am especially thinking of incurable cancer patients, of unsavable tuberculosis patients, of mortally wounded people, no matter where or how.

I find that having to face unbearable pain is absolutely unnecessary for the need for a death wish to arise. The painless hopelessness deserves equal sympathy.

It is also completely immaterial, whether under different circumstances the sick person could have been saved, since those more favorable conditions did not happen. "Unsavable" is also not meant in an absolute sense, but rather as beyond salvation in the concrete situation. When two friends go together on a dangerous mountain hike in a very remote area, one has a bad fall and breaks both his legs but the other cannot remove him, can also not call for or otherwise get help, then the suffering one is lost beyond salvation. If he realizes that and begs the friend for death, then the latter cannot resist and, if he is not weak, would also not want to resist him even at the personal risk of punishment. In the battlefield there are plenty of such cases. For people to do the right and dignified thing–there is no punishment for that and there should also be no threat of it either!

However, an absolutely necessary premise is not only the conviction of the consent or of the desire, but also the correct understanding [of the situation] by both parties, and not simply an hypochondriac assumption of the unsavable situation, but rather the mature assessment of the situation, of what life would be like for the one wishing to die.

The consent of the "incompetent" (German Civil Code § 104) is never enough. And a large number of additional "consents" must be considered equally insignificant. On the other hand, there are noteworthy consents also from minors still under the age of 18, and even from the insane as well.

When these unsavable people, whose life has become an unbearable burden, do not pass on suicide but rather – which can be very inconsistent, but may happen more frequently than not–beg for death by a third hand, there may be reasons for an inner contradiction, often to be found in the physical impossibility of suicide, due to the physical weakness of the sick person, to the unattainability of killing means, maybe even to the fact that the person is under surveillance or that he may be prevented from attempting suicide, but often also simply because of pure weakness in will power.

I can find absolutely no reason, from a legal, social, moral, religious point of view, not to allow those that want it, to kill those beyond salvation, who desperately desire it: I rather consider this concession simply as a responsibility of legal compassion, as it is already often applied in other ways. The essentials of the form of the execution will be discussed later.

However, how does this fit with considerations for the feelings, maybe even the strong interests, of the relatives with respect to the continuation of this life? The wife of the sick person, who loves him passionately, clings to his life. Maybe he maintains his family through his pension, in which case, this [action] would most highly contradict the act of mercy.

It should however emerge here that compassion for those beyond salvation must absolutely outweigh any other considerations. Also, nobody expects his loved ones to help him carry his mental anguish. He cannot do anything for them; he causes them daily new pain, which may perhaps be hard for them to endure; he must decide whether he still wants to carry on with this lost life. It is not possible to grant a right to object or an impediment right for the relatives–always with the assumption that the death wish is a significant one.

2. The second group consists of incurable idiots–either whether they were born that way or whether they became that way in the last phase of their suffering as a paralytic.

They have neither the will to live, nor to die. Therefore, from their point of view, there is no significant consent to the killing, but, on the other hand, the latter [action] does not infringe on any will to live that would have to be broken. Their life is totally without purpose, but they do not see it as unbearable. Their life produces a terribly heavy load for the relatives and for society. Their death does not create the smallest gap–except maybe in terms of the mother's feelings or those from the caring nurse. Since they require greater care, they justify the reason to establish a profession, which arises from the prolongation of a total unworthy life over years and decades.

There is no denying the fact that this contains a terrible contradiction, a misuse of life for its unworthy purpose.

Again, I can find absolutely no reason, from a legal, social, moral, religious point of view, to give permission for killing these people, which comprise the dreadful counterpart to real people and quickly arouse horror in nearly anyone (obviously, not *everyone*) that encounters them! In times of higher morals–ours have lost any heroism–these poor people would be officially liberated from themselves. These days, however, who would venture to confess this need, and therefore this permission, in our unnerved times? And therefore it should be asked today: who should be allowed to perform this killing? I would think that the relatives, who care for him, and whose life is constantly so heavily burdened by his existence, should be the first, even when the person being cared for has been placed in an institution, and next would be their legal guardians–depending on whether the former or the latter apply for the permission.

It is hardly possible to give this right to apply to the head of the mental institute. I would also think that the mother, who could not deny her love to her child despite the circumstances, should be allowed to object, in the event that she takes care for the child herself or pays for the care. It would be by far best, if the request was made as soon as the incurable idiocy was diagnosed.

3. I have spoken of a middle group and I find it in the mentally sane people, who have become unconscious through any kind of event, for instance a very serious, undoubtedly fatal injury, and who, if they ever were to regain consciousness, would wake up to a nameless misery.

As far as I know, these unconscious states can last so long, that it is no longer possible to speak of the assumption of an accidental case of euthanasia. But in most of the cases in this group, they should still be allowed to exist. Then the principle that was developed above (Ch. II, Pg. 6-7) comes full circle.

Regarding what little is left, it should still be noted: here too the possible consent of the unsavable in the killing is missing–even though due to totally different reasons compared to those for the mentally retarded . If this [action] was however taken arbitrarily with the belief that the victim would have given his consent to the killing, if only he had been able to, then, out of compassion, the executor runs a higher risk of sparing the unconscious [person] from a terrible end rather than robbing him of his life.

I do not think that it is possible to put forth handling standards for this group of killings. Instances will come up where the killing appears objectively justified; however, we may also be reminded that the person in question has become the offender in a rush under the assumption of doing the right thing. In that case, he would never be guilty of a deliberate illegal action, but may still be guilty of involuntary manslaughter.

For the killing that is later recognized to be justified, the legal option should be made available to let it go unpunished.

In conclusion, the only people that are being considered to be allowed to be killed are still always only the sick beyond salvation, where the unsavable condition has always to be combined with the desire or consent to be killed, or it would be, if the sick person had not reached the critical point in time of unconsciousness, or if he were ever able to regain awareness of his condition.

As already expressed above, any permission to the killing is ruled, if it were to go against the will to live of the person to be killed or already killed.

The permission to kill anybody is equally ruled out–I want to use for once the dreadful expression of a *prosciptio bona mente*.

The same way that permission to carry out the suicide can only be given to a single person, permission to kill those beyond salvation can only be given to those, who, based on the circumstances, would [otherwise] be called in to save them, and whose act of compassion can therefore find the understanding of all human beings displaying the appropriate feelings.

To clearly legally define the circle of these people is impossible. Whether the applicant and the executor of the permission in the individual case belong to this circle can only be determined on a case by case basis.

The relatives will often, but by no means all the time, belong to this circle. Hatred can surely take on the mask of compassion and Cain beat his brother Abel to death.

V. The Decision Over Allowing [the Act of Killing].

It is possible that the suggestions of the expansion of the areas of unprohibitive killings were met with full approval, at least in their first theoretical part, and that however their practical impossibility to be carried out prevented them from being put forth in the field.

It can be said with good reason: the assumption of allowing the act of killing is always formed on the pathological condition of prolonged terminal illness or incurable mental retardation. This condition requires a more objective professional statement, which cannot possibly be left in the hands of the executor. It would be however very easy to think that someone had a bigger interest, possibly even property rights, in the passing away of the sick person, and successfully sought out the agreement of the caring physician in the deadly intervention, or that the latter decided for himself, based on insufficient dialogue, to play out the fate.

If one now looked at the chosen case (above Ch. III, IV 1-3) under a different light, then a larger difference is apparent, after which the deadly interference becomes acutely necessary, after enough time for the preliminary examination of its assumptions. This time is always given for the second group (Ch. III, IV 2 incurable idiots), also surely sometimes for the third group after longer continuous unconsciousness, and, in a larger number of cases, for the first group–whether this group is predominantly larger, it remains debatable. It is however necessary to put forth the requirement, when it is feasible without skipping the necessary time for careful preliminary examination, that this preliminary examination also be carried out in as fast a process as possible, and that the decision be made immediately.

The process with mandatory preliminary examination must also be considered, as far as possible, as without exception.

The first question is then how to practically set it up, and then, what is to be done with those poor unsavable people and with those, who want to liberate them out of compassion, if the opportunity for an official preliminary examination is not given?

1. Permission From a State Authority.

Since today's State can never take the initiative itself to such killings, then initiation [for allowing such acts] will

1. be transferred to specific people entitled to make the request in the form of a petition for permission. For the first group, this can be the terminally ill himself, or his doctor, or anyone else whom he has entrusted with the position of making the request, especially one of his next of kin.

2. This request goes to a state authority. Its first job consists uniquely of determining the prerequisites to grant the permission: these consist of establishing the incurable nature of the illness or incurable nature of idiocy, and eventually, in the case of the first group, determining the ability of the sick person to provide an informed consent.

Their occupation should be stated: a doctor for an illness of the body, a psychiatrist or a second doctor, who is entrusted with the mentally ill, and a jurist that looks out at the law. These alone have a right to vote. It would be appropriate to perform this decision-making concerning the permission with a chairman who runs the negotiation but has no right to vote. Because, if any one of the former three people were entrusted with the chairman position, then he would be more powerful in the group compared to the other two, and that would not be desirable. A unanimous consent must be reached in order to grant the permission. The petitioner and the patient's doctor cannot be members of the committee.

This authority must be granted the right to visual inspection and witness examination.

3. The decision itself shall only state that, after careful examination of the conditions of the sick person, he appears incurable based on the current scientific view, if applicable, that there is no doubt about the validity of his informed consent, that there is no reason that stands in the way of the appropriate killing of the sick person, and that the petitioner is entrusted to put in motion in the proper way the liberation of the ill from his suffering.

Nobody shall be granted a right to kill, far less a duty to kill–not even the petitioner. The execution act must be the product of free compassion for the sick. The sick person, who has formally declared his consent, can obviously take it away at any moment and, with that, also [take away] the prerequisite for allowing the killing, so that the permission is therefore subsequently obviously overturned.

It can be recommended, based on the conclusion from the findings of the individual case, that in this case suitable means for euthanasia can be described. That the relief must be absolutely painless, and only an expert would be entitled to the use of the means.

4. A very careful protocol on the act of the execution would be delivered.

2. Arbitrary Killing of an Incurable Person Under the Assumption That the Prerequisites for Allowing the Killing Have Been Met.

This route, while in accordance with regulations, is however not always feasible. Maybe its representation is not even conceivable. Maybe even the time, which would cost him greatest hastening, would expose the incurably sick to unbearable suffering.

Then one has the alternative: either uncompassionately leave the incurable to continue in their suffering till the end due to practical difficulties and let his relatives and doctor remain fully passive despite their compassion, or do not forbid these "involved parties" to run the risk of making sure for themselves whether the prerequisites for the non-punishable killing apply, and to act in their best conscience based on the findings.

I do not hesitate for a single moment to speak out in favor of the second alternative.

In the event, then, that an incurable person was killed, in order to liberate him–be it with his consent, be it under the assumption that the sick person would have consented without any doubt and is only prevented from doing so by his state of unconsciousness–then, in my opinion, the legal option should be made prominent for such an executor and his helpers to go unpunished, and they would remain unpunished if the prerequisites of the permission are later proved to have been in place.

An "explanation duty" would be imposed for such cases, i.e. a duty to report about his action immediately after its execution to the allowing committee.

Otherwise, he could possibly be charged with involuntary manslaughter, as already ruled in the Prussian Common Law: The executor has mistakenly considered the prerequisites for his nonpunishable killing to be in place. This is not a true case of intent to destroy a life.

Therefore, based on our suggestions, there would be two new forms of unprohibited killing of third parties: the execution of the expressly allowed killing and the arbitrary killing under the correct assumption that the prerequisites for allowing it are met in the specific case through a person entitled to submit a request.

VI. Considering the Possibility of an Erroneous Permission.

In the case of the latter form, the executor runs the risk of making a mistake and even incurs the punishment on account of an unforgivable mistake.

It would, however, be received particularly badly by popular patrols, if a killing was caused by an erroneous official permission. For that exact reason, it is unavoidable to express an objection to our suggestions, as the diagnosis of incurability is uncertain and therefore the official permission could also be to the disadvantage of the person, who could maybe still eventually have been saved by a "miracle" or the doctor's skills. Such an event would however be most objectionable.

The possibility of a mistake by the department that allows these actions is, despite the required unanimity, undeniable. It can be quickly excluded only for the permanently mentally retarded. But mistakes are possible in all human actions, and nobody will make the foolish demand, that all useful and salutary actions should be stopped in view of this possible fault. Even the doctor outside the office can make a mistake, which can cause very bad consequences, and nobody will want to eliminate him because of his ability to make mistakes.

The good and the reasonable must happen despite any risks of mistakes.

Now, if during the course of cases with incorrect action, enough evidence of a mistake is supplied to make it obvious, the proof for the alleged mistake [committed] by the allowing department dare only be very difficult to provide and hardly increase to the level of a possibility of the assumption of survival.

Even accepting for once that the mistake took place, now humanity counts one less life. This life could have maybe still been very valuable after successfully overcoming the catastrophe: in most cases, however, it would have hardly had more than average value. The loss is obviously very hard for the relatives. However, humankind looses so many relatives due to mistakes, that one more or less really makes hardly any difference on the scale.

And would the preservation have always been a blessing for those saved from a serious disease? Maybe he would have still suffered deeply from the consequences of the severe illness; maybe he would have later met with a bad fate; maybe he would have had a very bad death: now he has however–at least at the moment–gently passed away.

His achieved life's rest shall be considered as a not-excessive price for the liberation of so many that cannot be saved from their sufferings.

In his so valuable paper on suicide, Gaupp talks about (Pg. 24) a catatonic, who had shot himself eleven times, where one of the bullets had remained in the brain and four others in the cranium.

"After being confined to bed for a long time, he recovered from his wounds, only to fall into a deep stupor, from which he woke up feeble-minded."

A dreadful testimonial of our times! We concentrate our efforts, with an endless expenditure of time, and patience and worry, to preserve lives with negative values, for which any reasonable person should hope for their passing. Our compassion rises above its right measure into cruelty. Not to allow a gentle death to the incurable, who longs for it, that is no longer compassion, but rather its opposite.

Also, a mistake, and maybe even a bad end, is still possible by all other actions of compassion. Who, however, wants to see the use of this very best trait of human nature restricted through the hint of such a mistake?

II.

Medical Remarks

by
Professor U. Hoche, M.D., Freiburg (in Breisgau).

The points discussed above through legal explanations do not all require an equal elucidation from a medical point of view. The question about the legal nature of suicide and the legal condition of the killing of the consenting victim shall not occupy us any longer; everything else, however, concerns us doctors–professionally occupied with the whole chain of thought of punishable or nonpunishable intervention in a foreign life–very much. The doctor's behavior towards killing in general [is an integral part of his profession], and it therefore requires a special discussion.

It is generally known that every person is justified, under legal closely defined circumstances, to unpunished interference in another's bodily existence (self-defense, desperate situation); for doctors, the negative behavior towards other people's lives is actually determined by law; as a matter of fact, the doctor's behavior in this area is a result of his special medical ethics. Usually, the general public is hardly aware of the fact that these medical moral teachings are not recorded anywhere. There are most likely individual books on the topic, which are however unknown to most doctors and portray purely elective procedures of their author, but there is no moral law in the paragraphs of medical lives, no "moral (civil) service regulations"

The young doctor goes straight on with his practice without every legal transcription of his rights and duties with respect to the points of intervention. The doctor's oath of earlier days with agreed general commitments is no longer available. What the novice brings with him in terms of instruction, is the example of his teachers at the university, the occasional discussions, which are linked to the individual case, the learning during his resident years, the influence of the general medical views from the literature, and his personal conclusions, which he draws from the uniqueness of his job. On certain topics, but just not the decisive ones, a decision is passed through the industrial code, contracts with the health insurance company and the likes; somewhat from a distance, the doctor sees some paragraphs of the penal code and receives supervision from his colleagues through the medical professional tribunal. All these cases, however, are mostly about a negative obligation for the doctor with respect to what he may not do, and not about positive instructions. What he may and should do results from the product of the currently accepted views, of which it is a prerequisite under all conditions, that the doctor is obliged to act based on general moral standards; consequently, the standing duty of his job is to heal the sick, to eliminate or alleviate pain, to retain and, as much as possible, to prolong life.

This general rule is not without exception. The doctor is practically required to destroy life (killing the live child at birth in order to save the mother, interrupting the pregnancy for the same reasons). These interventions are never expressly allowed; they only remain unpunished based on the view that they are in the interest of securing a higher legal asset and under the prerequisites that they have run out of all mandatory considerations, that all rules were followed in the execution, and that the necessary understanding has taken place with the patient or his legal representative or the next of kin.

Even the acts of body injury, as the surgeon undertakes as a profession and specialty, are never expressly allowed. They only remain unpunished when the rules were followed with respect to proof of need and careful execution. Therefore, a certain percentage of deadly outcomes is tacitly calculated into all surgical operations, where the highest efforts of medical skills are employed to reduce this number to a minimum, but which can however never be completely eliminated, resulting in turn also in cases, in which a human life is destroyed as a result of medical action. Our sense of morality has had to resign itself to this completely. The higher legal interest in the recovery of the majority makes the sacrifice of a minority necessary, where, in the individual case, the reassurance of the necessity of the preceding provision is given in the consent of the sick or their legal representative to the intervention, whose prerequisite is, as a rule, that the doctor has explained to him to the best of his knowledge the level of probability of his recovery, as well as the dangers to his life.

Also, with the exception of the above-mentioned type of questions, the doctor often faces the problem of an intervention into a life in a morally doubtful situation.

The wish "that they want it to be over soon" is not rarely expressed by the relatives in cases of terminal illness or incurable mental defects.

Just recently, the relatives of a suicide victim in a deep coma, who was the "black sheep" of the family, requested that I rather not do anything to resuscitate her. It can also happen, that the family, in the heat of the moment, holds it against the doctor, when the latter refuses to actively shorten that lost and possibly painful life. Nevertheless, it is a bigger step to go from this instinctive impulse all the way to the resolution to kill, or even just to [receive] the explicit consent from the family; based on human nature, the doctor, who is now being pressured by the relatives into shortening a life, would later in no way be safe from vehement reproach or even criminal charges.

The doctor can also be occasionally tempted, under very specific conditions, to interfere with human life out of a scientific interest. I remember such a temptation during my resident years, which I was triumphantly able to overcome in the end. A child with a rare and scientifically interesting brain disease was going to die and the condition was such, that he was surely going to die within the next 24 hours. If the child died in the hospital, we would have been able to perform an autopsy and take the desired look at the diseased brain. On the other hand, the father seemed to have the pressing desire to take the child home; if that was the case, we would lose the chance to perform the autopsy, which would otherwise be guaranteed, if the death occurred right before the collection. It would have been easy, and could not have been proven in any way, if at the time I had sped up the death, which was so absolutely sure, by a few hours through a morphine injection. In the end, I did not do anything, because my personal desire after scientific knowledge did not offer me enough rights to weigh against the medical duty not to shorten any life.

How one can decide, in such a case, whether for instance in the above-depicted circumstances, it would have been possible to later rescue innumerable human lives based on the far-reaching insight that could have been gained [from this action], this would be a new question, which should rather be answered from a higher standpoint.

Put in another way, the doctor has often to deal with the inner dilemma, when faced with the question of whether he should facilitate death by passively letting it happen, by avoiding the appropriate intervention, in cases where the patient willingly wishes to leave this life and has in any way put himself in a seriously dangerous situation through his attempt to commit suicide.

The temptation, in such cases, to let fate run its course, is then especially great when it is the case, for instance, of incurable mental patients, for whom death is in any case preferable.

(Obviously this whole dilemma does not apply in the case of certain illnesses, like for instance in the case of a simple curable depression, of a temporary erroneous assessment in the evaluation of the pressing need to die.)

This short list of cases, all of which I can speak of from personal experience, shows how tremendously complicated the consideration between the rigid principles of medical standards and the demands of a higher view of the value of life can already be in the daily life of the doctor. The doctor has no absolute, but rather only a relative connection with the fundamentally recognized task of preserving other people's lives under all circumstances; a connection, which changes under new circumstances and needs to be newly reevaluated. The medical ethics are not to be seen as an eternally unchangeable object. Historic progress shows us enough significant changes in this respect. From the moment on, when for instance the killing of the unsavable or the elimination of the mentally dead were to be recognized and accepted not only as not punishable but rather as a desirable goal for the general welfare, then in any case there would be no lack of objections to be found in the medical ethics.

For instance, doctors would find it to be a liberation of their conscience, when they were no longer restricted and oppressed in their handling of the dying by the categorical rule of the absolute prolongation of life, a rule, which I have also adopted–*de lege lata*–in my above-mentioned remarks; I would love to be allowed to change that sentence: "it used to be an essential demand..." The life-prolonging interventions planned by the doctors (or, on their orders, by the nursing staff and by the relatives) towards the dying, which are done for them and which should be a positive thing for them, are in reality a multiple evil, an annoyance, an ordeal, in the same way that the disruption of constant waking up is for the healthy, tired, sleeping patients; in by far the majority of the cases, the layman has the wrong idea about the inner conditions of the dying, whose awareness is either obscured in a salutary way, or who by now, after being worn down for a long time by pain and other inconveniences of his disease, only has the re-

31

maining desire for peaceful and quiet sleep and surely feels no gratitude towards anybody that inhibits and delays his always deeper sinking into unconsciousness; in truth, he is no longer capable of recognizing the good intention behind the disruptive care interventions.

Taken to the extreme, the recognized principle of the medical responsibility of prolonging life as much as possible, becomes nonsense; "A good deed turns into a plague". The main objection to my medical statement regarding the correct execution shall form the answer to the above-formulated question: "Is there a human life that has lost so clearly the quality of legal protection, that its continuation has permanently lost any value for both the person in question and for society?"

In general, this question must first be answered affirmatively with conviction; as far as the individual cases, the following is to be said. The legal component of the creation of the two groups that belong to these cases corresponds with the actual circumstances; the overall point of view of the worthless life summarizes however something very diversified; for the first group of those lost beyond salvation through disease or injury, their subjective and objective life value is not always equally lifted, while in the case of the second, also much larger, group of the incurable idiots, the continuation of life itself has no value for either the person in question or society.

With regards to the finality of incurable idiocy or, as we want to put it in more friendly terms: with regards to mental death, this is for instance fairly common for the doctor, especially for the nut doctor and the neurologist.

For practical purposes, they are divided into two large groups:

1. in those cases, in which, after a foreseeable time, mental death would have acquired full mental value or at least averageness in the later course of the life;

2. in those case, which have arisen due to brain changes established at birth or in early childhood.

32

It must be mentioned for the non-medical reader, that in the first group the circumstance for a mental death are reached: by changes of the brain through aging, then by the so-called softening of the brain in layman's terms, the *Dementia paralytica*, further more by the changes in the brain caused by arteriosclerosis, and finally by the large group of the dulling processes of people's minds (*Dementia praecox*), of which however only a certain percentage reaches the highest level of mental dulling of the mind.

The second group consists of either serious deformities of the brain, missing of individual parts (of larger or smaller areas), of developmental inhibitions during growth in the mother's womb, which can still carry an effect during the first years of life, or of disease processes during early childhood, which arrest normal development of the brain; (often these are associated with epileptic seizures or other motor dysfunctions).

Both groups can be left in equally high levels of mental stupor. For our purposes, however, it is still necessary to consider a difference, a difference in the state of mental stock, which is comparatively the same, as [the difference] between a pile of rocks lying around without any order, which have not yet been touched by a molding hand, and the rock debris of a collapsed building. In general, the expert is capable of making the distinction between the former and the latter conditions, even without knowledge of the history of a mentally dead person and without bodily examination, simply based on the picture of the mental defect.

Also, there is an essential difference left to be considered as far as the connections that the two different forms of mental death have established with the environment. For those that acquired the condition very early, they never achieved a mental rapport with their surroundings; for those that acquired it late, this was maybe possible in adequate measure. Therefore, the environment, the relatives and friends have a totally different relation to this subjective view of the latter; mentally dead people of this kind may have acquired a completely different "affection value"; there are feelings of pity, of gratitude towards them; numerous memories, maybe colored by strong emotions, are tied to their images, and all of this continues even when the emotions of the healthy environments no longer provoke any response from the sick person.

For this reason, a different measuring stick needs to be used for the question of any destruction of unworthy lives from the ranks of the feeble-minded, depending on whether they belong to the former or the latter category.

Also, with respect to the scientific and moral burden on the environment, the mental institution, the state, etc, the feeble-minded are never worth the same. The smallest burden on this front is given by the cases of brain softening of one form or another, for which, from the moment that they occur, it is truly possible to speak of complete mental death, and have in general only still a few years (at most) to live. A little more leeway can be found in cases of geriatric idiocy. Those suffering from mental atrophy caused by youth processes can, under the right circumstances, still live in this condition for another 20 or 30 years, while in cases of complete idiots based on very early changes it is a matter of an entire lifetime and, with that, the need of external care from two generations so that he can grow up.

From an economic point of view, these complete retards, just as they meet from very early on all the prerequisites to be classified as fully mentally dead, they would also be at the same time those, whose existence weighs heaviest on society.

The burden is partly of a financial nature and can be calculated based on the preparation of the annual balance sheet from the mental institution. I had this compiled for me, through a request to the German official institution in question to procure me the needed material. It results from that, that the median expenditure per head and year for the care of the retarded amounts so far to 1,300 million. When we add up the number of mentally retarded that were at the same time in the care of an institute in Germany, then we roughly come up with a total number of about 20-30,000. If we consider a median lifespan of 50 years for the single case, then it is easy to comprehend what an enormous capital–in terms of nourishing means, clothing and heating–is diverted from the national assets towards an unproductive purpose.

This is however by no means where the real burden is expressed.

The institutions, which care for the idiots, are deprived of other purposes; as long as these are private institutions, the interest return needs to be calculated; care personnel of several thousand heads is tied up for this completely unfruitful task and overbearing job; it is an embarrassing idea, that whole generations of caregivers grow old next to these empty human shells, several of whom live to be 70 or older.

The question of whether the necessary expenditure for these categories of cumbersome existence is justified at any cost, was not a pressing one in the past years of prosperity; now things are different, and we must seriously deal with it. Our situation is the same as that of participants in a difficult expedition, for which the biggest possible performance of everybody is the essential prerequisite for the success of the enterprise, and for which there is no room for half-, quarter- or eighth-strengths. For a long time, the task of us Germans is going to be: the most highly intensified aggregation of all possibilities, the liberation of all available power for more productive purposes. Modern endeavors stand in the way of the fulfillment of this task, endeavors to also retain all weaklings of all sorts at any cost, all of them, also even those that are not quite mentally dead, but who are still granted care and protection by their organization from elements of inferior quality–efforts, which retain this way their special scope, that so far it has not been possible, even really not seriously attempted, to prevent these people from reproducing.

It is going to remain tremendously difficult for a long time to attempt to somehow sort out these things in a legislative way, and also the thought of relieving our national overburdening by allowing the destruction of the completely worthless and mentally dead is going to meet first, and maybe still for a long time, against lively, predominantly instinctive objections, which are going to draw their strength from very different sources (dislike for the new, religious beliefs, sentimental feelings and so on). In an examination focused on reaching of the most likely tangible outcome, as is the case for the one in front of us, this point must therefore be handled in the form of the theoretical discussion of the possibilities and conditions, not however in that of the "request".

In all cases of worthlessness as a result of mental death there is a contradiction between their subjective rights on existence and objective usefulness and necessity.

Up until now, the nature of the solution to this conflict was the measuring stick for the level of attained humanity in the individual human cycles and in the individual domains of this world, to which today's standard has taken a longer, more tiring developmental road, partly under the essential collaboration of the Christian set of ideas.

Seen from the point of view of a higher civil morality, there is no doubt that exaggerations are being exercised in the striving for the absolute preservation of unworthy life. We have learned, from someone else's point of view, to consider in this respect the state organism as a whole with its own laws and rights, in the same way as, for instance, it would be for a self-contained human organism, which, as us doctors know, surrenders and rejects individual parts or particles that have become worthless or damaged in the interest of the well-being of the whole.

An overview of the series of ballast existences presented above and a short reflection show that the majority of them does not come into consideration for the question of a conscious rejection, i.e. disposal. We never want to stop taking care of deficiencies and infirmities also in times of need, which we are facing now, as long as they are not mentally dead; we will never stop treating bodily and mentally sick people to the utmost, as long as there is still any chance of improvement in their condition; we may however one day mature to the view that the *disposal of the fully mentally dead does not represent any violation, any immoral act, any instinctive brutality, but rather an allowable useful act.*

Here, we are first interested in the question of which qualities and actions befit the conditions of mental death. A superficial connection is without further due noticeable: the foreign nature of the body of the mentally dead within the structure of human communities is a condition of complete helplessness, which requires care by third parties and lacks any productive contribution.

With respect to the inner condition, the term of mentally dead would include that no clear ideas, feelings or intentions can be created based on the condition of the brain, that there is no awareness of any chance of revival of a world view, and that there can be no emotional connections going out from the mentally dead towards the environment, (even if they may well be the object of affection from third parties).

The most important [part], however, is the lack of the possibility to become aware of their own personality, the lack of self-awareness. The mentally dead possess an intellectual level, which we first find at the very bottom of the animal chain, and also the emotions that they feel do not rise above the bar of the most elementary processes, which are associated with animal life.

Therefore, a mentally dead person is also not capable of raising an inner subjective claim to life, just as poorly as he would be capable of other mental processes.

This latter point only appears to be unnecessary; in truth, it has its meaning in the sense that the disposal of a mentally dead person cannot be equated to any other death.

37

From a purely legal point of view, the destruction of a human life already never means the same.

The differences do not only lie in the motives of the killing, (depending on: murder, manslaughter, negligence, self-defense, duel, etc.), but also in the behavior of the person being killed towards their claim to life. While the deliberately planned killing of another against their will (premeditated murder) carries the death penalty, the killing from a death-wish of the victim is handled with just a few years in prison. The act of interference in someone else's life is actually the same in each case. If there was any doubt on the matter, the killing as a consequence of a desire by the victim is actually a colder, more systematic, carefully thought-out action than murder, and yet it is lumped together with much lesser crimes because the person to be killed had given up their subjective claim to life and, in contrast, invoked his right to death.

(Nothing should be changed in this analysis also for the curable mental patients, who have no subjective claim to life, or who, in contrast, make even energetic claims towards its destruction, but earn no consideration whatsoever in their desire to die because they suffer from morbid motives of a periodic nature; these cases are incidentally far away from the condition of mental death.)

In the case of the killing of a mentally dead person, who, based on the way things are due to the condition of his brain, is not capable of making a subjective claim on anything at all, including, among other things, to levy on life, consequently no subjective claim can be violated.

It can therefore be concluded, also without adding anything else on the topic concerning the inner mental condition of the mentally dead, that it is wrong to apply the viewpoint of compassion to them; the mistake, which underlies the compassion for the worthless life, is the deep-rooted flaw in reasoning, or rather lack of reasoning, by dint of which the majority of people project their own thinking and feelings onto the other person's life, and which is also one of the sources of the rise in animal cults among Europeans. "Compassion" towards the mentally dead either in life or in case of death is at the bottom of the list of appropriate feelings; Where there is no suffering, there is also no "co-suffering"[30].

Despite all this, only a very slow process of conversion and resetting is going to be possible for this new question. The awareness of the loss of meaning of the individual existence, as measured in relationship to the interest of the whole, the feeling of an absolute duty to gather all available energies and reject all unnecessary tasks, the feeling of being the most responsible accomplice of a heavy undertaking full of suffering, all of this will have to become common view on a much larger scale compared to what it is today, before the view presented here can receive full recognition. Human beings are in general capable of bigger and stronger emotions only under special exceptions and always only for a short time; for this reason, special single activities in this direction make such a big impression. We read with dramatic compassion about the account of Greeley's polar expedition, of how he was forced, in order to increase the chances of survival of the community, to let one of the members, who did not stick to the rationing and thus became a danger to all through his unauthorized eating, be shot in the back, since his resolve had been reconsidered by all; it fills us with legitimate compassion, when we read how Capt. Scott and his followers, on the way back home from the South Pole, made the difficult sacrifice in the interest of saving the life of the others, that one member would willingly leave the tent and freeze to death outside in the snow.

30

      The term "compassion" is derived from the two Latin words "*com*" (with) and "*pati*" (to suffer). The term used by the author in the original manuscript ("Mitleid"), is a literal translation of those two word, i.e. mit= with, Leid=suffering), so that the author can use this in a play of words to make his point across (***TN***)

A small part of such heroic soul feeling must humble us, before we can approach the complications of the theoretical possibilities discussed here.

In the end, everything that deals with the connection to our portrayal of the necessity of technical guarantees against erroneous or misused actions, is object of medical evaluation.

To being with, the idea will naturally arise, that the complications of the extreme thought that has been expressed here may open the door for criminal misuse. In light of the constant mistrust that the common citizen displays towards the many legislations that somehow interfere in their private existence, here too possibilities storm in and are lead into the field. It is the same line of thought and feelings, which effortlessly jumps to the conclusion that it would be a small thing for the wealthy to be capable of acquiring a medical certificate of mental incompetency in criminal cases, which makes it believable and possible for the lay person, that medical certificates would attest to their mental incapacity, which would appear believable and probable to the layman, resulting in constant internment of the mentally sane and legal incapacitations from profit-seeking relatives, views, which have no less been thickened by the practical legislative inappropriateness, which had been reduced, in the question of legal incapacitation, to the right of application by the state attorney in his time (by alcoholism).

The guarantee against such opinions would be found in a carefully treated technique.

With this respect, it is up for debate, whether the selection of the cases, which have become permanently worthless for both the individual in question as well as for society, can be made with such certainty, as to exclude any mistakes and errors.

This can only be a concern for the lay person. For the doctor, there is not the slightest doubt, that this selection can be carried out with 100% certainty, meaning therefore with a completely different measure of certainty as for instance for the question of whether it can be decided if executed criminals are mentally sane or mentally insane.

The doctor has numerous scientific, and without a doubt more amenable, criteria at his disposal, from which he can recognize the impossibility of improvement of a mentally dead person, so much more so, since the former youth suffering from mental death is at the forefront in consideration for our entire problem.

Obviously, no doctor will want to already declare with certainty a two or three year old child as permanently mentally dead. It arrives the time, however, still during childhood, when this future determination can be met without any doubt.

The formation of a qualified committee for the most accurate examination of the situation has already been discussed in the legal part of this manuscript. I am also convinced, despite the overtone of fruitlessness, which we innerly hear at the mention of the word "committee", that the establishment of such an organization would be necessary. I find the discussion of the details less pressing than the belief that obviously the prerequisite for the realization of this train of thought must be the development of all thinkable guarantees in any direction.

The image of the development of more important human questions, which he later sensualizes in a spiraling form, comes from Goethe. The crux of this image is the fact that a spiral line that runs upwards along a trunk, always comes back to the same side of the trunk and passes on at known distances, but each time a stock higher.

This image will also later show itself in this cultural question of ours. There was a time, which we now view as barbaric, in which the disposal of those born with unlivable conditions was considered natural, and then came the still on-going phase, in which the preservation of any whatsoever worthless existence is ultimately considered the highest moral requirement; there will be a new age, which, from the point of view of a higher morality, will stop making heavy sacrifices on the basis of an exaggerated concept of humanity and an over-protection of the value of mere existence. I know that today these explanations will find by no means approval, or even just understanding, everywhere; this point of view should not induce those, who can speak up from a right based on more than a generation of medical human services, to be silent.

DIE FREIGABE DER VERNICHTUNG LEBEN-SUNWERTEN LEBENS

Ihr Maß und ihre Form.

Ich darf bekunden, daß die Fragen, mit denen unsere Abhandlung sich be schäftigt, dem Verstorbenen Gegenstand eines von lebhaftestem Verantwortungsgefühl und tiefer Menschenliebe getragenen Nachdenkens gewesen sind.

Mir persönlich wird die Erinnerung an die Stunden der gemeinsamen Arbeit mit dem Feuerkopf voll kühlscharfen Verstandes immer ein wehmütig stimmender Besitz bleiben.

Freiburg i. Br., den 10. April 1920.

Hoche.

I.
Rechtliche Ausführung
von
Professor Dr. jur. et. phil. Karl Binding.

Ich wage am Ende meines Lebens mich noch zu einer Frage zu äußern, die lange Jahre mein Denken beschäftigt hat, an der aber die meisten scheu vorübergehen, weil sie als heikel und ihre Lösung als schwierig empfunden wird, so daß nicht mit Unrecht gefragt werden konnte, es handle sich hier "um einen starren Punkt in unseren moralischen und sozialen Anschauungen".

Sie geht dahin: soll die unverbotene Lebensvernichtung, wie nach heutigem Rechte - vom Notstand abgesehen -, auf die Selbsttötung des Menschen beschränkt bleiben, oder soll sie eine gesetzliche Erweiterung auf Tötungen von Nebenmenschen erfahren und in welchem Umfange?

Ihre Behandlung führt uns von Fallgruppe zu Fallgruppe, deren Lage jeden von uns aufs tiefste erschüttert. Um so notwendiger ist es, nicht am Affekt, andererseits nicht der übertriebenen Bedenklichkeit das entscheidende Wort zu überlassen, sondern es auf Grund bedächtiger rechtlicher Erwägung der Gründe für und der Bedenken gegen die Bejahung der Frage zu finden. Nur auf solch steter Grundlage kann weiter gebaut werden.

Ich lege demnach auf strenge juristische Behandlung das größte Gewicht. Gerade deshalb kann den festen Ausgangspunkt für uns nur das geltende Recht bilden: wieweit ist denn heute - wieder vom Notstande abgesehen - die Tötung der Menschen *freigegeben*, und was muß denn darunter verstanden werden? Den Gegensatz der "Freigabe" bildet die Anerkennung von Tötungrechten.

Diese bleiben hier vollständig außer Betracht.

Die wissenschaftliche Klarstellung des positivrechtlichen Ausgangspunktes aber ist um so unumgänglicher, als er sehr häufig falsch oder doch sehr ungenau gefaßt wird.

I. Die heutige rechtliche Natur des Selbstmordes.
Die sog. Teilnahme daran.

I. Von einer Macht, der er nicht widerstehen kann, wird Mensch für Mensch ins Dasein gehoben. Mit diesem Schicksale sich abzufinden - das ist seines Lebens Besitz. Wie er dies tut, das kann innerhalb der engen Grenzen seiner Bewegungsfreiheit er nur selbst bestimmen. Insoweit ist er der geborene Souverän über sein Leben.

Das Recht - ohnmächtig dem Einzelnen die Tragkraft nach der ihm vom Leben auferlegten Traglast zu bestimmen - bringt diesen Gedanken scharf zum Ausdruck durch Anerkennung von jedermanns Freiheit, mit seinem Leben ein Ende zu machen. Nach langer höchst unchristlicher Unterbietung dieser Anerkennung - von der Kirche gefordert, gestützt auf die unreine Auffassung, der Gott der Liebe könnte wünschen, daß der Mensch erst nach unendlicher körperlicher und seelischer Qual stürbe, - dürfte sie heute - von ganz wenigen zurückgebliebenen Staaten abgesehen - wieder voll zurückgewonnener, für alle Zukunft unangefochtener Besitz bleiben.

Das Naturrecht hätte Grund gehabt, von dieser Freiheit als dem ersten aller "Menschenrechte" zu sprechen.

II. Wie diese Freiheit aber gesehen werden muß im Rahmen unseres politischen Rechtes, dies steht noch keineswegs fest. Ebenso in falscher Terminologie, als in falschen praktischen Folgerungen spricht sich diese Unsicherheit aus. Es ist höchste Zeit, daß größte wissenschaftliche Genauigkeit die bisherige ungenaue Behandlung der einschlagenden Fragen ablöse -, daß insbesondere die fundamentale rechtliche Verschiedenheit zwischen dem schlecht sog. Selbstmord und der Tötung Einwilligender klar erkannt werden.

Zwei sich im tiefsten widersprechende Auffassungen vom Selbstmord gehen heute nebeneinander her -

beide übereinstimmend nur darin, daß sie falsch sind, und daß sie auf dem Postulat seiner Straflosigkeit münden.

I. Nach der einen ist der Selbstmord widerrechtliche Handlung, Delikt, qualitativ dem Mord und dem Totschlag aufs engste verwandt, weil Übertretung des Verbotes der Menschentötung.

Solche Ausdehnung der Tötungsnorm ist unseren gemeinrechtlichen Quellen ganz fremd, und alle Beweise für die deliktischen Eigenschaften des Selbstmordes versagen. Alle religiösen Gründe besitzen für das Recht aus doppeltem Grunde keine Beweiskraft. Sie beruhen hier auf ganz unwürdiger Gottesauffassung, und das Recht ist durch und durch weltlich: auf Regelung des äußeren menschlichen Gemeinlebens eingestellt. Nebenbei gefragt, berührt das neue Testament das Problem mit keinem Wort.

Die gleiche Urkraft, für die Rechtswidrigkeit des Selbsttötung zu beweisen, eignet der ebenso haltlosen als "pharisäischen" (Gaupp) Behauptung, sie sei stets eine unsittliche Handlung und so verstehe sich ihre Rechtswidrigkeit von selbst.

Schon der "harte und lieblose" Name Selbstmord für die eigene Tötung ist tendenziös. Denn dem "Morde" waren stets feige Heimlichkeit und Niedertracht wesentlich. Und nun bedenke man zunächst die große Anzahl psychisch gestörter Personen, die Hand an sich legen! Außerdem gibt es altruistische Selbsttötungen geistig völlig Gesunder, die auf der höchsten Stufe der Sittlichkeit stehen, andererseits Selbsttötungen, die bis auf den tiefsten Grad frivoler Gemeinheit oder elender Feigheit herabsinken können. Ja es gibt unterlassene Selbsttötungen, die gerade wegen der Unterlassung schweren sittlichen Tadel verdienen.

Außerdem ist die sittliche Handlung als solche durchaus nicht auch rechtswidrig und die rechtmäßige durchaus nicht immer sittlich.

Der Beweis der Widerrechtlichkeit der Selbsttötung könnte nur aus dem exakten Nachweis der positivrechtlichen Tötungsnorm geführt werden. Dafür fehlt aber das Material überall, wo die Selbsttötung nicht unter Strafe gestellt oder sonst unzweideutig als Delikt gekennzeichnet ist. Oder sie könnte sich als Folgerung aus rechtlich feststehenden Prämissen ergeben. Solchen Nachweis versuchte Feuerbach aber in der unzulänglichsten Weise. " Wer in den Staat eintritt — der Neugeborene tritt aber doch nicht ein ! —, verpflichtet dem Staat seine Kräfte und handelt rechtswiedrig, wenn er ihm diese durch Selbstmord eigenmächtig raubt". Das ist offenbar eine nichtssagende petitio principä.

So fehlt für die Deliktsnatur der Selbsttötung nicht nur alles Beweismaterial, sondern es fällt auch heutzutage keinem Selbstmörder und keinem seiner Beurteiler auch nur von ferne ein, in der Selbsttötung eine verbotene Handlung zu erblicken und diese wirklich qualitativ auf eine Linie mit Mord und Totschlag zu stellen.

Wer aber die Deliktsauffassung vertritt, der muß unter allen Umständen die sog. Teilnehmer an der Selbsttötung unter der Voraussetzung verschuldeten Handelns gleichfalls als Delinquenten betrachten. Und aus der Straflosigkeit des Selbstmörders ist die der "Teilnehmer" dogmatisch gar nicht ohne weiteres zu folgern: denn sie handeln widerrechtlich gegen das Leben eines Dritten, stehen somit auf höherer Stufe der Strafbarkeit als der, der sich nur an sich selbst vergreift, wenn dessen Tat als Delikt betrachtet wird.

In Konsequenz der Auffassung von der Deliktseigenschaft der Selbsttötung hätten die Staatsorgane, zu deren Aufgabe die Deliktshinderung gehört, ein Zwangsrecht zur Unterlassung der Tötung gegen den Selbstmörder und seine sog. Teilnehmer, wogegen diesen Allen natürlich ein Notwehrrecht nicht zustünde.

Ganz naturrechtlich gedacht, wenn auch durchaus nicht immer von den durch die kirchliche Auffassung stark beeinflußten Naturrechtslehrern vertreten, ist die entgegengesetzte Auffassung: die Selbsttötung ist die Ausübung eines Tötungsrechtes. Auch sie findet in den Quellen nicht die geringste Stütze: denn die Straflosigkeit des Selbstmordes kann als solche nicht betrachtet werden. Es gibt straflose Delikte in Fülle. So ist sie eine rein theoretische Konstruktion, die sich einer vollständigen Verkennung des Wesens der subjektiven Rechte und der üblichen Verwechslung der Reflexwirkung von Verboten mit solchen Rechten schuldig macht. Da die Tötung nur des Nebenmenschen verboten ist, so wird gefolgert, hat jeder Mensch ein Recht entweder auf Leben oder am Leben oder gar über das Leben - alle drei Auffassungen sind gleich verkehrt -, und kraft dieses Besitzrechtes darf er das Leben ebenso behaupten als von sich wehren, besitzt er also ein Tötungsrecht an sich selbst oder wider sich selbst, ja kann dieses vielleicht gar mit Bezug auf sich selbst auf andere übertragen.

Lasse ich das ganz unmögliche Recht auf oder am oder über das eigene Leben einmal auf sich beruhen - ganz gut dagegen E. rupp S. 15 -, so ist gegen das Selbst-Tötungsrecht einzuwenden, daß Handlungsrechte nur zu Zwecken verliehen werden, welche der Rechtsordnung generell als ihr konform, ihr förderlich erscheinen. Darin liegt also eine generelle Billigung der Handlung von Rechts wegen. Solche verbietet sich jedoch gegenüber der Selbsttötung unbedingt. Übt diese doch in einer nicht kleinen Zahl ihrer Vorkommnisse auf dem Rechtsgebiet sehr empfindliche schädliche Wirkungen aus: etwa die Begründung weitgehender öffentlicher Unterstützungspflichten. Ja, sie kann geradezu das Mittel zur Verletzung schwerer Rechtspflichten bilden: etwa der Pflichten, keine Schulen zu bezahlen, keine Strafe zu verbüßen, an gefährlicher Stelle vor dem Feinde Vorpostendienste zu leisten oder einen Angriff mitzumachen.

Stellt man sich aber einmal auf diesen Standpunkt

der Anerkennung von der Rechtmäßigkeit der Selbsttötungshandlung, so ergibt sich

a.) daß niemand ein Recht besitzen kann, den Selbstmörder an seiner rechtmäßigen Tat zu hindern;

b) daß diesem gegen jeden Hinderungsversuch ein Notwehrrecht zusteht;

c) daß, wenn man das Recht des Menschen sich selbst zu töten gar als ein übertragbares betrachtet, alle sog. Teilnehmer, die mit seiner beachtlichen Einwilligung handeln - aber allerdings nur diese -, gleichfalls rechtmäßig handeln, also gleichfalls daran von niemandem gehindert werden dürfen und gegen jeden Hinderungsversuch die Notwehr besitzen.

Alle Teilnehmer jedoch, die ohne solche Einwilligung handeln, versieren in re illicita, dürfen, ja müssen eventuell an Ausführung ihrer Handlung gehindert werden, und machen sich im Schuldfall grundsätzlich verantwortlich.

Ja, vom Standpunkt dieses übertragbaren Tötungsrechtes aus muß sogar

d) die Tötung des beachtlich Einwilligenden gleichfalls als rechtmäßige Tötungshandlung betrachtet werden.

III. Läßt sich der Selbstmord weder als eine deliktische noch als eine rechtmäßige Handlung auffassen, so bleibt nur übrig, ihn als eine rechtlich unverbotene Handlung zu begreifen. Diese Auffassung, die freilich in recht verschiedener Formulierung mehr und mehr durchdringt, findet eine verschiedene Begründung, welche Verschiedenheit hier auf sich beruhen bleiben kann. Ich habe mich früher darüber so ausgesprochen: dem Rechte als der Ordnung des menschlichen Gemeinschaftslebens "widerstrebe die Scheidung von Rechtssubjekt und Rechtsobjekt auf das Individuum zu übertragen und dieses einem Dualismus untertan zu machen, wonach es auch für sich selbst Güterqualität, vielleicht gar Sachenqualität annehmen muß, damit es Rechte an sich selbst und Rechtspflichten wider sich selbst erlangen könne."

Es bleibt eben dem Rechte nichts übrig, als den lebenden Menschen als Souverän über sein Dasein und die Art desselben zu betrachten. Daraus ergeben sich sehr wichtige Konsequenzen:

1. Diese Anerkennung gilt nur dem Lebensträger selbst. Nur seine Handlung gegen sich selbst ist unverboten.

2. Diese Anerkennung stellt keine Ausnahme vom Tötungsverbot dar; denn dieses unterfragt nur die Tötung des Nebenmenschen, und daraus folgt eben das Unverbotensein der Selbsttötung.

3. Alle sog. Teilnahme am Selbstmord unterfällt der Tötungsnorm, ist also widerrechtlich, kann, ja muß unter Umständen unter Strafe genommen werden, falls es nicht, was möglich ist, an der Schuld fehlt. Das "kann" besagt: de lege ferenda, das "muß" besagt: de lege lata, falls der sog. Teilnehmer Mittäter oder Urheber ist.

4. Nur die Handlung des Verstorbenen ist unverboten. Ganz ohnmächtig ist er, durch seine Zustimmung auch die Handlungen Dritter zu unverbotenen zu gestalten. Mit allerbestem Grunde betrachtet unser positives Recht die Tötung der Einwilligenden als Delikt.

5. Ist ihm die Handlung unverboten, so darf ihn niemand daran hindern, wenn er genügend weiß, was er tut; gegen den Hindernden hat er dann das Notwehrrecht; der Zwang gegen ihn, die Handlung zu unterlassen, ist rechtswidrige Nötigung.

Diese Erretter vom Selbstmord handeln meist optima fide und gehen dann straflos aus. Eine starke Stütze für ihren Standpunkt bildet die Erfahrung, daß der gerettete Selbstmörder oft sehr glücklich über seine Rettung ist und den zweiten Versuch nach dem mißlungenen ersten meist unterläßt.

IV. Der rechtlich und sozial schwache Punkt der Freigabe aller Selbsttötung ist der Verlust der ganzen

Anzahl noch durchaus lebenskräftiger Leben, deren Träger nur zu bequem oder zu feig sind, ihre durchaus tragbare Lebenslast weiter zu schleppen.

Es fällt dies für die Wertung der Schuld der sog. Teilnehmer stark in die Waagschale. Die bewußte Beihilfe zum Selbstmord des Todkranken wiegt erheblich leichter wie die zu dem der Gesunden, der sich etwa seinen Gläubigern entziehen will.

II. Keiner besonderen Freigabe bedarf die reine Bewirkung der Euthanasie in richtiger Begrenzung.

Scheinbar und für eine rein kausale Betrachtung ganz zweifellos eine Tötung Dritter, welche bisher nach meiner Kenntnis strafrechtlich noch nicht verfolgt worden ist, bildet die Herbeiführung der sog. Euthanasie.

I. Der in der neueren Literatur aufgetauchte unschöne Name der "Sterbehilfe" ist zweideutig. Völlig außer Betracht muß hier das schmerzstillende Mittel bleiben, das die wirkende Todesursache der Krankheit in ihrer Wirkung beläßt. Allein bedeutsam wird für unsere Betrachtung die Verdrängung der schmerzhaften, vielleicht auch noch länger dauernden, in der Krankheit wurzelnden Todesursache durch eine schmerzlosere andere. Einem am Lungenkrebs furchtbar schwer Leidenden macht der Arzt oder ein anderer Hilfsreicher eine tödliche Morphiuminjektion, die schmerzlos, vielleicht auch rascher, vielleicht aber auch erst in etwas längerer Zeit den Tod herbeiführt.

II. Um die rechtliche Natur dieser Handlung, ihre Rechtswidrigkeit oder ihr Unverbotensein - denn von einem subjektiven Recht ihrer Vornahme kann unmöglich gesprochen werden - ist derselbe m. E. ganz unnötige Streit entstanden wie über die Natur des ärztlichen - richtiger des auf Heilung abzielenden - scheinbaren Eingriffs in die Gesundheit, besonders in die Körperintegrität eines anderen.

Die Lage, in welcher diese Handlung der Bewirkung von Euthanasie vorgenommen wird, muß aber genau präzisiert werden: dem innerlich Kranken oder dem Verwundeten steht der Tod von der Krankheit oder der Wunde, die ihn quält, sicher und zwar alsbald bevor, so daß der Zeitunterschied zwischen dem infolge der Krankheit vorauszusehenden und dem durch das untergeschobene Mittel verursachten Tode nicht in Betracht fällt. Von einer spürbaren Verringerung der Lebenszeit der Verstorbenen kann dann überhaupt nicht oder höchstens nur von einem beschränkten Pedanten gesprochen werden.

Wer also einem Paralytiker am Anfang von dessen vielleicht auf die Dauer von Jahren zu berechnenden Krankheit auf dessen Bitte oder vielleicht sogar ohne diese die tödliche Morphiumseinspritzung macht - bei dem kann von reiner Bewirkung der Euthanasie keine Rede sein. Hier ist eine starke, auch für das Recht ins Gewicht fallende Lebensverkürzung vorgenommen worden, die ohne rechtliche Freigabe unzulässig ist.

III. In demselben Augenblick aber wird klar: die sichere Ursache qualvollen Todes war definitiv gesetzt, der baldige Tod stand in sichere Aussicht. An dieser toddrohenden Lage wird nichts geändert, als die Vertauschung dieser vorhandenen Todesursache durch eine andere von der gleichen Wirkung, welche die Schmerzlosigkeit vor ihr voraus hat. Das ist keine "Tötungshandlung im Rechtssinne", sondern nur eine Abwandelung der schon unwiderruflich gesetzten Todesursache, deren Vernichtung nicht mehr gelingen kann: es ist in Wahrheit eine reine Heilhandlung. "Die Beseitigung der Qual ist auch Heilwerk."

Als verbotene Tötung könnte solch Verhalten nur betrachtet werden, wenn die Rechtsordnung barbarisch genug wäre zu verlangen, daß der Todkranke durchaus an seinen Qualen zugrunde gehen müsse. Davon kann doch zur Zeit keine Rede mehr sein.

Es ist beschämend, daß man je daran hat denken, je danach hat handeln können!

IV. Daraus ergibt sich: es handelt sich hier gar nicht um eine statuierte Ausnahme von der Tötungsnorm, um eine rechtswidrige Tötung, falls von dieser nicht eine Ausnahme ausdrücklich anerkannt worden wäre, sondern um unverbotenes Heilwerk von segensreicher Wirkung für schwer gequälte Kranke, um eine Leidverringerung für noch Lebende, solange sie noch leben, und wahrlich nicht um ihre Tötung.

So muß die Handlung als unverboten betrachtet werden, auch wenn das Gesetz ihrer gar nicht im Sinne der Anerkennung Erwähnung tut.

Und zwar kommt es dabei auf die Einwilligung des gequälten Kranken gar nicht an. Natürlich darf die Handlung nicht seinem Verbot zuwider vorgenommen werden, aber in sehr vielen Fällen werden momentan Bewußtlose Gegenstand dieses heilenden Eingriffes sein müssen. Aus der Natur dieser Handlung ergibt sich auch, daß die Beihilfe zu ihr und die Bestimmung dazu seitens eines Dritten gleichfalls durchaus unverboten sind. Die irrtümliche Annahme der Tödlichkeit der Lage kann den zur Bewirkung der Euthanasie Verschreitenden wegen fahrlässiger Tötung verantwortlich machen.

III. Ansätze zu weiterer Freigabe.

Unsere Anfangsuntersuchung hat ergeben: unverboten ist heute ganz allein die Selbsttötung in vollstem Umfange. Von einer Freigabe der sog. Teilnahme daran ist zurzeit gar keine Rede. Denn in allen Formen ist sie deliktischer Natur. Auch durch die Einwilligung des Selbstmörders kann sie davon nicht entkleidet werden. Aber zufolge der verkehrten akzessorischen Behandlung der sog. Teilnahme im Gesetzbuch wird bewirkt, daß die Beihilfe zum Selbstmord straflos bleiben muß, und in der vorsätzlichen Bestimmung zum Selbstmord seine Anstiftung zur demselben im Sinne des § 48 des GB. gefunden werden darf - einerlei ob der Selbstmörder zurechnungsfähig ist oder nicht.

Eine weitere Freigabe könnte also nur eine Freigabe der Tötung des Nebenmenschen sein. Sie würde bewirken, was die Freigabe des Selbstmordes nicht bewirkt: eine echte Einschränkung des rechtlichen Tötungsverbotes.

Für eine solche ist neuerdings verschiedentlich eingetreten worden, und als Stichwort oder Schlagwort für diese Bewegung wurde der Ausdruck von dem Recht auf den Tod geprägt.

Darunter ist nicht sowohl ein echtes Recht auf den Tod verstanden, sondern es soll damit nur ein rechtlich anzuerkennender Anspruch gewisser Personen auf Erlösung aus einem unerträglichen Leben bezeichnet werden.

Diese neue Bewegung ist vorbereitet durch zwei Strömungen, deren eine, die radikalere, sich durchaus in dem Gebiet der aprioristischen wie der gesetzauslegenen Theorie, die andere, ängstlichere und zrückhaltendere, sich in dem der Gesetzgebungen gebildet hat.

I. Es ist bekannt, daß die Römer die Tötung des Einwilligenden straflos gelassen haben. Auf Grund ganz übertreibender Deutung der I. 1 § 5 D de injuriis 47, 10: quia nulla injuria est, quae in voentem fit, die sich lediglich auf das römische Privatdelikt der injuria bezog, wurde nun wieder die ganz naturrechtliche Lehre ausgebildet von der ungeheuren Macht der Einwilligung des Verletzten in die Verletzung. Diese schließe durchweg, wenn überhaupt von einem der Tragweite dieser Einwilligung Bewußten erteilt, soweit es bei Delikten überhaupt einen Verletzten gebe, die Rechtswidrigkeit der Verletzung aus: die Handlung könne also gar nicht gestraft werden, jede Verletzung des Einwilligenden, insbesondere sein Tötung, sei unverbotene Handlung.

Auf diesen Standpunkt stellten sich im vorigen Jahrhundert W. v. Humboldt (Gesamm. W. VII S. 138), Henke und Wächter, später besonders Ortmann, Rödenbeck, Keßler, Klee, E. Rupp. Bleiben sie konsequent, so müssen sie energische Gegner des GB. § 216 werden.

II. Die Begegnung innerhalb der Gesetzgebung knüpft gleichfalls an die Einwilligung in die Verletzung an, die im Interesse ihrer klareren Erkennbarkeit und leichteren Beweisbarkeit zum Verlangen der Verletzung gesteigert wurde.

Dieses Verlangen der Tötung wird zum Strafmilderungsgrund, die Tötung auf Verlangen bleibt also echtes Verbrechen - Verbrechen natürlich nicht im Sinn des SRtGB. § 1 genommen.

Es hat damit begonnen das Preußische Landrecht T. II Tit. 20 § 834. Viele deutschen Strafgesetzbücher sind ihm gefolgt, aber nicht schon das Bayrische v. 1813, sondern zuerst das Sächsische v. 1838. Auch das Preußische verhielt sich ablehnend, ebenso von seinen Nachfolgern das Oldenburgische v. 1858 und das Bayrische v. 1861, nicht aber das Lübische (f. § 145).

Es zwang diese Abweisung des Verlangens des Strafmilderungsgrundes zu dem furchtbar harten Schluß, die Tötung des Einwilligenden der Strafe des Mordes oder des Totschlages zu unterstellen.

Diese unerträgliche Notwendigkeit hat denn auch dazu geführt, in den dritten Entwurf des Norddeutschen

Strafgesetzbuchs - die beiden ersten hatten wirklich geschwiegen! - die Tötung des den Tod ausdrücklich und ernstlich Verlangenden seitens dessen an den das Verlangen gerichtet war, als selbständiges Tötungs-"Vergehen" aufzunehmen und deshalb unter die im Mindestbetrag noch viel zu hohe Gefängnisstrafe von nicht unter 3 Jahren zu stellen. Dieser Vorschlag hat dann unverändert Aufnahme in das Gesetz gefunden. Es liegt dem das richtige Verständnis eines notwendig anzuerkennenden Strafmilderungsgrundes unter.

Die Tötung des Einwilligenden hat nicht nötig den Lebenswillen des Opfers zu brechen, durch welche Vergewaltigung die regelmäßige Tötung erst ihre furchtbare Schwere erlangt.

Darin liegt der Zwang, den Deliktsgehalt der Tötung des Einwilligenden zunächst als objektiv bedeutend geringer zu fassen. Damit wird auf der subjektiven Seite eine Abmilderung der Schuld dann Hand in Hand gehen, wenn die Handlung aus Mitleiden verübt wird. Aber notwendig ist dies zur Strafmilderung gar nicht - weder nach theoretischem Gesichtspunkte, noch de lege lata. Indessen weiter als zur Strafmilderung führt die zum Verlangen gesteigerte Einwilligung in die Tötung de lege lata nicht.

Der rechtlich schwachen Punkte dieser privilegierten Art vorsätzlicher Tötung sind drei: 1. die gesetzliche Steigerung der Einwilligung zum Verlangen oder gar zum ausdrücklichen Verlangen zwingt, die Tötung des nicht in dieser gesteigerten Form Einwilligenden auch wieder als Mord oder gewöhnlichen Totschlag zu behandeln;

2. das Gesetz unterscheidet nicht zwischen Vernichtung des lebenswerten und lebensunwerten Lebens;

3. das Gesetz erweist seine Wohltat auch dem sehr grausam Tötenden. - Den zweiten dieser Mängel hat aber eine Anzahl unserer Strafgesetzbücher klar erkannt.

Fünf unserer früheren Strafgesetzbücher, zuerst das

Württembergische v. 1839 (U. 239), kennen ein doppelt privilegiertes Tötungsverbrechen: nämlich die Tötung auf Verlangen vollführt an "einem Todkranken oder tödlich Verwundeten".

Hier bricht klar der Gedanke durch, daß solch Leben den vollsten Strafschutz nicht mehr verdient, und daß das Verlangen seiner Vernichtung rechtlich eine größere Beachtung zu finden hat, als das Verlangen der Vernichtung robusten Lebens.

Dieser sehr gute Anfang hat jedoch im Reichsstrafgesetz keinen Fortgang, dagegen in der Literatur sehr lebhafte Aufnahme gefunden!

IV. Steigerung der Privilegierungsgründe des Tötungsdeliktes zu Gründen für die Freigabe der Tötung Dritter?

Bedenkt man, daß eine ganze Anzahl namhafter Juristen die Einwilligung in die Tötung deren Rechtswidrigkeit überhaupt ganz aufheben lassen, somit die Tötung des Einwilligenden jedenfalls als unverboten behandelt sehen wollen, daß andererseits in neuerer Zeit von edlem Mitleid mit unertragbar leidenden Menschen stark bewegte und erfüllte Stimmen für Freigabe der Tötung solcher laut geworden sind, so muß man doch wohl behaupten: es stünde zurzeit de lege ferenda doch zur Frage, ob nicht der eine oder der andere dieser beiden Strafmilderungsgründe zu einem Strafausschließungsgrund erhoben oder ob nicht mindestens beim Zusammentreffen der beiden Privilegierungsgründe: Einwilligung und unterträglichen Leidens die Tötung als gerechtfertigt, will sagen als unverboten betrachtet werden solle?

Es ist nicht uninteressant zu sehen, daß die Verfasser des Vorentwurfes von 1909 die Privilegierung dessen unbedingt ablehnen, "der einen hoffnungslosen Kranken ohne dessen Verlangen aus Mitleiden des Lebens beraube".

Wie rückständig sind diese Gesetzgeber der Gegenwart hinter dem Preußischen Landrecht geblieben, das Teil II Lit. XX § 833 für die damalige Zeit so großherzig und zugleich juristisch so fein bestimmt hat: "Wer tödlich Verwundeten, oder sonst Todkranken, in vermeintlich guter Absicht, das Leben verkürzt, ist gleich einem fahrlässigen Totschläger nach § 778.779 zu betrafen." Die angedrohte Strafe ist sehr mild: Gefängnis oder Festung "auf einen Monat bis zwei Jahre".

Über hundert Jahre sind seitdem ins Land gegangen, und solch köstliche Satzung hat für das deutsche Volk keine Frucht getragen! Das Norwegische Strafgesetzbuch v. 22. Mai 1902 § 235 hat die Strafbarkeit solcher Tötung der der Tötung des Einwilligenden gleichgestellt. Die Motive des deutschen Entwurfs von 1909 führen aus: solche Vorschrift könne "in schlimmer Weise mißbraucht und das Leben erkrankter Personen in erheblicher Weise gefährdet werden", auch sei eine befriedigende Fassung dafür kaum zu finden.

I. Ich will nun für den Augenblick einmal beide Fäden abreißen, um sie später wieder anzuknüpfen, vor allem Weiteren aber die Vorfrage stellen, die gegenwärtig m. E. unbedingt gestellt werden muß. Die juristische, scheinbar so geschäftsmäßige Formulirung scheint auf große Herzlosigkeit zu deuten: in Wahrheit entspringt sie nur dem tiefen Mitleiden.

Gibt es Menschenleben, die so stark die Eigenschaft des Rechtsgutes eingebüßt haben, daß ihre Fortdauer für die Lebensträger wie für die Gesellschaft dauernd allen Wert verloren hat?"

Man braucht sie nur zu stellen und ein beklommenes Gefühl regt sich in Jedem, der sich gewöhnt hat, den Wert des einzelnen Lebens für den Lebensträger und für die Gesamtheit auszuschätzen. Er nimmt mit Schmerzen wahr, wie verschwenderisch wir mit dem wertvollsten, vom stärksten Lebenswillen und der größten Lebenskraft erfüllten und von ihm getragenen Leben umgehen, und welch Maß von oft ganz nutzlos vergeudeter Arbeitskraft, Geduld, Vermögensaufwendung wir nur darauf verwenden, um lebensunwerte Leben so lange zu erhalten, bis die Natur - oft so mitleidlos spät - sie der letzten Möglichkeit der Fortdauer beraubt.

Denkt man sich gleichzeitig ein Schlachtfeld bedeckt mit Laufenden toter Jugend, oder ein Bergwerk, worin schlagende Wetter Hunderte fleißiger Arbeiter verschüttet haben, und stellt man in Gedanken unsere Idioteninstitute mit ihrer Sorgfalt für ihre lebenden Insassen daneben - und man ist auf das tiefste erschüttert von diesem grellen Mißklang zwischen der Opferung des teuersten Gutes der Menschheit im größten Maßstabe auf der einen und der größten Pflege nicht nur absolut wertloser, sondern negativ zu bewertender Existenzen auf der anderen Seite.

Daß es lebende Menschen gibt, deren Tod für sie eine Erlösung und zugleich für die Gesellschaft und den Staat insbesondere eine Befreiung von einer Last ist, deren Tragung außer dem einen, ein Vorbild größerer Selbstlosigkeit zu sein, nicht den kleinsten Nutzen stiftet, läßt sich in keiner Weise bezweifeln.

Ist dem aber so - gibt es in der Tat menschliche Leben, an deren weiterer Erhaltung jedes vernünftige Interesse dauernd geschwunden ist - dann steht die Rechtsordnung vor der verhängnisvollen Frage, ob sie den Beruf hat, für deren soziale Fortdauer tätig - insbesondere auch durch vollste Verwendung des Strafschutzes - einzutreten oder unter bestimmten Voraussetzungen ihre Vernichtung freizugeben? Man kann die Frage legislatorisch auch dahin stellen: ob die energische Forterhaltung solcher Leben als Beleg für die Unangreifbarkeit des Lebens überhaupt den Vorzug verdiene, oder die Zulassung seiner alle Beteiligenden erlösenden Beendigung als das kleinere Übel erscheine?

II. Über die notwendig zu gebende Antwort kann nach kühl rechnende Logik kaum ein Zweifel obwalten. Ich bin aber der festen Überzeugung, daß die Antwort durch rechnende Vernunft allein nicht definitiv gegeben werden darf: ihr Inhalt muß durch das tiefe Gefühl für ihre Richtigkeit die Billigung erhalten. Jede unverbotene Tötung eines Dritten muß als Erlösung mindestens für ihn empfunden werden: sonst verbietet sich ihre Freigabe von selbst. Daraus ergibt sich aber eine Folgerung als unbedingt notwendig: die volle Achtung des Lebenswillens aller, auch der kränksten und gequältesten und nutzlosesten Menschen.

Nach Art des den Lebenswillen seines Opfers gewaltsam brechenden Mörders und Totschlägers kann die Rechtsordnung nie vorzugehen gestatten.

Selbstverständlich kann auch gegenüber dem Geistesschwachen, der sich bei seinem Leben glücklich fühlt, von Freigabe seiner Tötung nie die Rede sein.

III. Die in Betracht kommenden Menschen zerfallen nun, soweit ich zu sehen vermag, in zwei große Gruppen, zwischen welche sich eine Mittelgruppe einschiebt.

1. die zufolge Krankheit oder Verwundung unrettbar Verlorenen, die im vollen Verständnis ihrer Lage den dringenden Wunsch nach Erlösung besitzen und ihn in irgendeiner Weise zu erkennen gegeben haben.

Die beiden oben erwähnten Privilegierungsgründe treffen hier zusammen. Ich denke besonders an unheilbare Krebskranke, unrettbare Phthisiker, an irgendwie und wo tödlich Verwundete.

Ganz unnötig scheint mir, daß das Verlangen nach dem Tode aus unerträglichen Schmerzen entspringt. Die schmerzlose Hoffnungslosigkeit verdient das gleiche Mitleid.

Ganz gleichgültig erscheint auch, ob unter anderen Verhältnissen der Kranke hätte gerettet werden können, falls diese günstigeren Verhältnisse sich eben nicht beschaffen lassen. "Unrettbar" ist also nicht in absolutem

Sinne, sondern als unrettbar in der konkreten lage zu verstehen. Wenn zwei Freunde zusammen in abgelgenster Gegend eine gefährliche Bergwanderung machen, der eine schwer abstürzt und beide Beine bricht, der andere aber ihn nicht fortschaffen, auch menschliche Hilfe nicht errufen oder sonst erlangen kann, so ist eben der Zerschmetterte unrettbar verloren. Sieht er das ein und erfleht er vom Freunde den Tod, so wird dieser kaum widerstehen können und wenn er kein Schwächling ist, selbst auf die Gefahr hin in Strafe genommen zu werden, auch nicht widerstehen wollen. Auf dem Schlachtfeld ereignen sich sicher analoge Fälle zur Genüge. Die Menschen vom richtigen und würdigen Handeln abzuhalten - dazu ist die Strafe nicht da und dazu soll ihre Androhung auch nicht verwendet werden!

Unbedingt notwendige Voraussetzung ist aber nicht nur die Ernstlichkeit der Einwilligung oder des Verlangens, sondern auch für die beiden Beteiligten die richtige Erkenntnis und nicht nur die hypochondrische Annahme des unrettbaren Zustandes und die reife Auffassung dessen, was die Aufgabe des Lebens für den den Tod Verlangenden bedeutet.

Die Einwilligung des "Geschäftsunfähigen" (BGB § 104) genügt regelmäßig nicht. Aber auch eine große Zahl weiterer "Einwilligungen" wird als unbeachtlich betrachtet werden müssen. Andererseits gibt es beachtliche Einwilligungen auch von Minderjährigen nocht unter 18 Jahren, ja auch von Wahnsinnigen.

Wenn diese Unrettbaren, denen das Leben zur unerträglichen Last geworden ist, nicht zur Selbsttötung verschreiten, sondern - was sehr inkonsequent sein kann, aber doch nicht selten sich ereignen mag - den Tod von dritter Hand erflehen, so liegt der Grund zu diesem inneren Widerspruch vielfach in der physischen Unmöglichkeit der Selbsttötung, etwa in zu großer Körperschwäche der Kranken, in der Unerreichbarkeit der Mittel zur Tötung, vielleicht auch darin, daß er überwacht wird oder am Versuche des Selbstmordes gehindert würde, vielfach aber auch in reiner Willensschwäche.

Ich kann nun vom rechtlichen, dem sozialen, dem sittlichen, dem religiösen Gesichtspunkt aus schlechterdings keinen Grund finden, die Tötung solcher den Tod dringend verlangender Unrettbarer nicht an die, von denen er verlangt wird, freizugeben: ja ich halte diese Freigabe einfach für eine Pflicht gesetzlichen Mitleids, wie es sich ja doch auch in anderen Formen vielfach geltend macht. Über die Art des Vollzugs wird später das Nötige zu sagen sein.

Wie sieht es aber mit der Rücksichtnahme auf die Gefühle, vielleicht gar auf starke Interessen der Angehörigen an der Fortdauer dieses Lebens? Die Frau des Kranken, die ihn schwärmerisch liebt, klammert sich an sein Leben. Vielleicht erhält er durch Bezug seiner Pension seine Familie, und diese widerspricht dem Gnadenakt auf das energischste.

Mit will jedoch scheinen, das Mitleid mit dem Unrettbaren muß hier unbedingt überwiegen. Seine Seelenqual ihm tragen zu helfen vermag auch von seinen Geliebten keiner. Nichts kann er für sie tun; täglich verstrickt er sie in neues Leid, fällt ihnen vielleicht schwer zur Last; er muß entscheiden, ob er dies verlorene Leben noch tragen kann. Ein Einspruchsrecht, ein Hinderungsrecht der Verwandten kann nicht anerkannt werden - immer vorausgesetzt, daß das Verlangen nach dem Tode ein beachtliches ist.

2. Die zweite Gruppe besteht aus den unheilbar Blödsinnigen - einerlei ob sie so geboren oder etwa wie die Paralytiker im letzten Stadium ihres Leidens so geworden sind.

Sie haben weder den Willen zu leben, noch zu sterben. So gibt es ihrerseits keine beachtliche Einwilligung in die Tötung, andererseits stößt diese auf keinen Lebenwillen, der gebrochen werden müßte. Ihr Leben ist absolut zwecklos, aber sie empfinden es nicht als unerträglich. Für die Angehörigen wie für die Gesellschaft bilde sie eine furchtbar schwere Belastung. Ihr Tod reißt nicht die geringste Lücke - außer vielleicht im Gefühl der Mutter oder der treuen Pflegerin. Da sie großer Pflege bedürfen, geben sie Anlaß, daß ein Menschenberuf entsteht, der darin aufgeht, absolut lebensunwertes Leben für Jahre und Jahrzehnte zu fristen.

Daß darin eine furchtbare Widersinnigkeit, ein Mißbrauch der Lebenskraft zu ihrer unwürdigen Zwecken, enthalten ist, läßt sich nicht leugnen.

Wieder finde ich weder vom rechtlichen, noch vom sozialen, noch vom sittlichen, noch vom religiösen Standpunkt aus schlechterdings keinen Grund, die Tötung dieser Menschen, die das furchtbare Gegenbild echter Menschen bilden und fast in jedem Entsetzen erwecken, der ihnen begegnet, freizugeben - natürlich nicht an Jedermann! In Zeiten höherer Sittlichkeit - der unseren ist aller Heroismus verloren gegangen - würde man diese armen Menschen wohl amtlich, von sich selbst erlösen. Wer aber schwänge sich heute in unserer Entnervtheit zum Bekenntnis dieser Notwendigkeit, also solcher Berechtigung auf?

Und so wäre heute zu fragen: wem gegenüber darf und soll diese Tötung freigegeben werden? Ich würde meinen, zunächst den Angehörigen, die ihn zu pflegen haben, und deren Leben durch das Dasein des Armen dauernd so schwer belastet wird, auch wenn der Pflegling in eine Idiotenanstalt Aufnahme gefunden hat, dann auch ihren Vormündern - falls die einen oder die anderen die Freigabe beantragen.

Den Vorstehern gerade dieser Anstalten zur Pflege der Idioten wird solch Antragsrecht kaum gegeben werden können. Auch würde ich meinen, der Mutter, die trotz des Zustandes ihres Kindes sich die Liebe zu ihm nicht hat nehmen lassen, sei ein Einspruch freizugeben, falls sie die Pflege selbst übernimmt oder dafür aufkommt. Weitaus am besten würde der Antrag gestellt, sobald der unheilbare Blödsinn die Feststellung gefunden hätte.

3. Ich habe von einer Mittelgruppe gesprochen und finde sie in den geistig gesunden Persönlichkeiten, die durch irgendein Ereignis, etwa sehr schwere, zweifellos tödliche Verwundung, bewußtlos geworden sind, und die, wenn sie aus ihrer Bewußtlosigkeit noch einmal erwachen sollten, zu einem namenlosen Elend erwachen würden.

Soviel ich weiß, können diese Zustände der Bewußtlosigkeit so lange dauern, daß von den Voraussetzungen zufälliger Bewirkung der Euthanasie nicht mehr die Rede sein kann. Aber in den meisten Fällen dieser Gruppe dürften diese doch vorhanden sein. Dann greift der Grundsatz durch, der oben s. II S. 14 - 18 entwickelt worden ist.

Bezüglich des wohl kleinen Restes ist aber zu bemerken: Auch hier fehlt - wenn auch aus ganz anderem Grunde wie bei den Idioten - die mögliche Einwilligung des Unrettbaren in die Tötung. Wird diese jedoch eigenmächtig vorgenommen in der Überzeugung, der Getötete würde, wenn er dazu imstande gewesen wäre, seine Zustimmung zur Tötung erteilt haben, so läuft der Täter bewußt ein großes Risiko aus Mitleid mit dem Bewußtlosen, nicht um ihm das Leben zu rauben, sondern um ihm ein furchtbares Ende zu ersparen.

Ich glaube nicht, daß sich für diese Gruppe der Tötungen eine Regelbehandlung aufstellen läßt. Es werden Fälle auftauchen, worin die Tötung sachlich als durchaus gerechtfertigt erscheint; es kann sich aber auch ereignen, daß er Täter übereilt gehandelt hat in der Annahme, das Richtige zu tun. Dann wird er nie vorsätzlich rechtswidriger, wohl aber eventuell fahrlässiger Tötung schuldig.

Für die nachträglich als gerechtfertigt anerkannte Tötung sollte gesetzlich die Möglichkeit eröffnet werden, sie straflos zu lassen.

Die Personen also, die für die Freigabe ihrer Tötung allein in Betracht kommen, sind stets nur die unrettbar Kranken, und zu der Unrettbarkeit gesellt sich stets das Verlangen des Todes oder die Einwilligung, oder sie würde sich dazu gesellen, wenn der Kranke nicht in dem kritischen Zeitpunkt der Bewußtlosigkeit verfallen wäre oder wenn der Kranke je zum Bewußtsein seines Zustandes hätte gelangen können.

Wie schon oben ausgeführt, ist jede Freigabe der Tötung mit Brechnung des Lebenswillens des zu Tötenden oder des Getöteten ausgeschlossen.

Ebenso ausgeschlossen ist die Freigabe der Tötung an Jedermann - ich will einmal den furchtbaren Ausdruck einer proscriptio bona mente gebrauchen.

Wie die Selbsttötung nur einer einzigen Person freigegeben ist, so kann die Tötung Unrettbarer nur solchen freigegeben werden, die sie nach Lage der Dinge zu retten berufen wären, deren Mitleidstat deshalb das Verständnis aller richtig empfundenen Menschen finden wird.

Den Kreis dieser Personen gesetzlich bestimmt zu umgrenzen, ist untunlich. Ob der Antragsteller und der Vollstrecker der Freigabe im einzelnen Falle dazu gehörten, kann nur für jeden Einzelfall festgestellt werden.

Die Angehörigen werden vielfach, aber keineswegs immer dazu gehören. Der Haß kann auch die Maske des Mitleides annehmen und Kain erschlug seinen Bruder Abel.

V. Die Entscheidung über die Freigabe.

Es wäre möglich, daß diese Vorschläge der Erweiterung des Gebietes unverbotener Tötung seis ganz, seis wenigstens in ihrem ersten Teile theoretische Billigung fänden, daß aber ihre praktische Undurchführbarkeit gegen sie ins Feld geführt würde.

Mit gutem Grunde könnte gesagt werden: Voraussetzung der Freigabe bildet immer der pathologische Zustand dauernder tödlicher Krankheit oder unrettbares Idiotentum. Dieser Zustand bedarf objektiver sachverständiger Feststellung, die doch unmöglich in die Hand des Täters gelegt werden kann. Wäre doch sehr leicht denkbar, daß irgendwer an dem frühzeitigeren Hinscheiden des Kranken ein großes, vielleicht gar vermögensrechtliches Interesse hätte, und den behandelnden Arzt zum tödlichen Eingreifen erfolgreich zu bestimmten suchte, oder daß dieser von sich aus beschlösse, auf ungenügende Dialoge hin das Schicksal zu spielen.

Vergegenwärtigt man sich nun die einschlagenden Fälle (oben s. III, IV 1 - 3) in ihrer Verschiedenheit, so zeigt sich ein großer Unterschied, je nachdem der tödliche Eingriff sich akut notwendig macht, ober genügende Zeit für die Vorprüfung seiner Voraussetzungen gelassen ist. In der zweiten Gruppe (s. III, IV 2 unheilbarer Blödsinn) wird diese Zeit stets gegeben sein, in der dritten, bei länger dauernder Bewußtlosigkeit wohl auch manchesmal, in der ersten in einer größeren Anzahl der Fälle - ob der überwiegend größeren, bleibt zweifelhaft. Man wird die Forderung aufstellen müssen, daß wenn es angängig ist, diese nötige Zeit sorgfältiger Vorprüfung ausgespart, daß aber auch diese Vorprüfung in möglichst beschleunigtem Verfahren erledigt, und der Beschluß sofort gefaßt wird.

Das Verfahren mit obligatorischer Vorprüfung muß, soweit möglich, als das ausnahmelose betrachtet werden.

Fragen wir zunächst, wie es zweckmäßig einzurichten wäre, und dann, was mit den armen Unrettbaren und mit denen wird, deren Mitleid sie erlösen möchte, wenn die Möglichkeit amtlicher Vorprüfung nicht gegeben ist?

1. Die Freigabe durch eine Staatsbehörde.

Da der Staat von heute nie die Initiative zu solchen Tötungen ergreifen kann, so wird die Initiative

1. in der Form des Antrags auf Freigabe bestimmten Antragsberechtigten zu überweisen sein. Das kann in der ersten Gruppe der tödlich Kranke selbst sein, oder sein Arzt, oder jeder andere, den er mit der Antragstellung betraut hat, insbesondere Einer seiner nächsten Verwandten.

2. Dieser Antrag geht an eine Staatsbehörde. Ihre erste Aufgabe besteht ganz allein in der Feststellung der Voraussetzungen zur Freigabe: das sind die Feststellung unrettbarer Krankheit oder unheilbaren Blödsinns und eventuell die der Fähigkeit des Kranken zu beachtlicher Einwilligung in den Fällen der ersten Gruppe.

Daraus dürfte sich ihre Besetzung ergeben: ein Arzt für körperliche Krankheiten, ein Psychiater oder ein zweiter Arzt, der mit den Geisteskrankheiten vertraut ist, und ein Jurist, der zum Rechten schaut. Diese hätten allein Stimmrecht. Zweckmäßig wäre, diesen Freigebungsausschuß mit einem Vorsitzenden zu versehen, der die Verhandlungen leitet, aber kein Stimmrecht besitzt. Denn würde eine jener drei Persönlichkeiten mit dem Vorsitz betraut, so würde sie im Kollegium mächtiger als die beiden anderen, und das wäre nicht wünschenswert. Zur Freigabe dürfte Einstimmigkeit zu erfordern sein. Der Antragsteller und der behandelnde Arzt des Kranken dürften als Mitglieder dem Ausschusse nicht angehören.

Dieser Behörde müßte das Recht des Augenscheins und der Zeugenvernehmung erteilt werden.

3. Der Beschluß selbst dürfte nur aussprechen, daß nach vorgenommener Prüfung des Zustandes des Kranken er nach den jetzigen Anschauungen der Wissenschaft alsunheilbar erscheint, eventuell daß kein Grund zum Zweifel an der Beachtlichkeit seiner Einwilligung vorliegt, daß demgemäß der Tötung des Kranken kein hindernder Grund im Wege steht, und dem Antragsteller

anheimgegeben wird, in sachgemäßer Weise die Erlösung des Kranken von seinem Übel in die Wege zu leiten.

Niemandem darf ein Recht zur Tötung, noch viel weniger jemandem eine Pflicht zur Tötung eingeräumt werden - auch dem Antragsteller nicht. Die Ausführungstat muß Ausfluß freien Mitleids mit dem Kranken sein. Der Kranke, der seine Einwilligung auf das Feierlichste erklärt hat, kann sie natürlich jeden Augenblick zurücknehmen, und dadurch die Voraussetzung der Freigabe und damit sie selbst nachträglich umstürzen.

Es dürfte sich empfehlen, im Anschluß an den Befund des Einzelfalles das in diesem Falle geeignete Mittel der Euthanasie zu bezeichnen. Denn unbedingt schmerzlos muß die Erlösung erfolgen, und nur ein Sachverständiger wäre zur Anwendung des Mittels berechtigt.

4. Über den Vollzugsakt wäre dem Freigebungsausschuß ein sorgfältiges Protokoll zuzustellen.

2. Eigenmächtige Tötung eines Unheilbaren unter Annahme der Voraussetzungen freizugebender Tötung.

Dieser ordnungsgemäße Weg ist aber nicht immer gangbar. Vielleicht läßt sich seine Vertretung nicht einmal denken. Vielleicht könnte auch die Zeit, die er selbst bei größter Beschleunigung kosten würde, den Unheilbaren unerträglichen Qualen aussetzen.

Dann steht man vor der Alternative: entweder mutet man wegen praktischer Schwierigkeiten dem Unrettbaren mitleidlos die Fortdauer seiner Qualen bis zum Ende und seinen Angehörigen oder seinem Arzte trotz ihres Mitleids volle Passivität zu, oder man untersagt diesen "Beteiligten" nicht, das Risiko zu laufen, sich über die Voraussetzungen unverbotener Tötung selbst zu vergewissern und auf Befund nach bestem Gewissen zu handeln.

Ich zögere nicht einen Augenblick, mich für die zweite Alternative auszusprechen.

Tötet dann jemand einen Unheilbaren, um ihn zu erlösen - seis mit seiner Einwilligung, seis in der Annahme, der Kranke würde sie zweifellos erteilen und sei daran nur durch seine Bewußtlosigkeit gehindert, - so müßte m. E. für solchen Täter und seine Gehilfen gesetzlich die Möglichkeit, sie straflos zu lassen, vorgesehen sein, und sie würden straflos zu bleiben haben, wenn sich die Voraussetzungen der Freigabe nachträglich als vorhanden gewesen ergeben würden.

Dem Täter würde für solche Fälle eine "Verklarungspflicht" aufzuerlegen sein, d. h. eine Pflicht, von seiner Tat sofort nach ihrer Begehung bei dem Freigabeausschuß Anzeige zu machen.

Anderenfalls hätte eventuell angemessene Strafe wegen fahrlässiger Tötung Platz zu greifen, wie sie ja schon das Preußische Landrecht angeordnet hat: der Täter hat ja die Voraussetzungen seiner unverbotenen

Tötung zu Unrecht als vorhanden angenommen. Von echtem Lebensvernichtungsvorsatz ist bei ihm nicht zu sprechen.

So gäbe es nach unseren Vorschlägen zwei neue Arten unverbotener Tötungen Dritter: den Vollzug der ausdrücklich freigegebenen Tötung und die eigenmächtige Tötung unter richtiger Annahme der Voraussetzungen der Freigabe im konkreten Fall durch einen Antragsberechtigten.

VI. Das Bedenken der möglicherweise irrtümlichen Freigabe.

Bei der zweiten Art trägt der Täter das Risiko des Irrtums und verfällt bei unverzeihlichem Irrtum sogar der Strafe.

Ganz besonders schwer würde aber in weiten Volksstreifen eine Tötung auf Grund irrtümlicher amtlicher Freigabe empfunden werden. Gerade deshalb wird unseren Vorschlägen unausbleiblich der Einwand entgegengehalten werden, die Diagnose der Unheilbarkeit sei unsicher, und so könnte die amtliche Freigabe auch erfolgen zuungunsten eines Menschen, den ein "Wunder" oder die Kunst der Ärzte doch vielleicht schließlich noch hätte retten können. Solcher Vorgang sei aber im höchsten Maße anstößig.

Die Möglichkeit des Irrtums bei der Freigabebehörde ist trotz der geforderten Einstimmigkeit unleugbar. Nur bei den dauernden Idioten dürfte er fast ausgeschlossen sein. Aber Irrtum ist bei allen menschlichen Handlungen möglich, und niemand wird die törichte Folgerung ziehen, daß alle nützlichen und heilsamen Handlungen in Anbetracht dieses möglichen Defekts zu unterbleiben hätten. Auch er Arzt außerhalb der Behörde unterliegt dem Irrtum, der sehr üble Folgen verursachen kann, und niemand wird ihn wegen seiner Fähigkeit zu irren ausschalten wollen.

Das Gute und das Vernünftige müssen geschehen trotz allen Irrtumsrisikos.

Während nun bei Laufenden von Fällen irrigen Handelns der Beweis des Irrtums nachher bis zur Evidenz zu erbringen ist, dürfte der Beweis für den angeblichen Irrtum der Freigabebehörde nur sehr schwer zu beschaffen und kaum über den Grad einer Möglichkeit der Annahme des Überlebens zu steigern sein.

Nimmt man aber auch den Irrtum einmals als bewiesen an, so zählt die Menschheit jetzt ein Leben weniger. Dies Leben hätte vielleicht nach glücklicher Überwindung der Katastrophe noch sehr kostbar werden können: meist aber wird es kaum über den mittleren Wert besessen haben. Für die Angehörigen wiegt natürlich der Verlust sehr schwer. Aber die Menschheit verliert infolge Irrtums so viele Angehörige, daß einer mehr oder weniger wirklich kaum in die Waagschale fällt.

Und wäre denn immer für den aus schwerer Krankheit Geretteten die Erhaltung ein Segen gewesen? Vielleicht würde er an den Folgen der schweren Erkrankung doch noch viel gelitten haben; vielleicht hätte ihn schweres Schicksal später geschlagen; vielleicht hätte er einen sehr schweren Tod gehabt: jetzt ist er - allerdings vorzeitig - aber sanft entschlafen.

Sein erhaltbar gewesener Lebensrest darf als ein nicht übertriebener Kaufpreis für die Erlösung so vieler Unrettbaren von ihren Leiden betrachtet werden.

In seiner so wertvollen Abhandlung über den Selbstmord berichtet Gaupp (S. 24) von einem Katatoniker, der sich elf Kugeln in den Körper geschossen habe, von denen eine ins Gehirn, vier andere im Schädel geblieben sind.

"Nach langem Krankenlager genas er von seinen Verletzungen, um weiterhin in einen tiefen stupor zu verfallen, aus dem er blöde erwachte."

Ein furchtbares Zeugnis unserer Zeit! Mit Aufwand

unendlicher Zeit und Geduld und Sorge bemühen wir uns um die Erhaltung von Leben negativen Wertes, auf dessen Erlöschen jeder Vernünftige hoffen muß. Unser Mitleiden steigert sich über sein richtiges Maß hinaus bis zur Grausamkeit. Dem Unheilbaren, der den Tod ersehnt, nicht die Erlösung durch sanften Tod zu gönnen, das ist kein Mitleid mehr, sondern sein Gegenteil. Auch bei allen anderen Handlungen des Mitleids ist der Irrtum und vielleicht auch ein übles Ende möglich. Wer aber möchte die Anwendung dieses schönsten Zuges menschlicher Natur durch den Hinweis auf solchen Irrtum beschränkt sehen?

II.

Ärztliche Bemerkungen

von
Professor Dr. U. Hoche, Freiburg i. Br.

Die von den vorausgehenden rechtlichen Ausführungen besprochenen Punkte bedürfen nicht alle in gleichem Maße einer Beleuchtung vom ärztlichen Standpunkte aus. Die Frage der rechtlichen Natur des Selbstmordes und der Rechtslage bei der Tötung der Einwilligenden soll uns nicht länger beschäftigen; alles andere aber geht uns Ärzte sehr viel an, durch deren Köpfe berufsmäßig die ganze Gedankenreihe strafbarer oder strafloser Eingriffe in fremdes Leben hindurchläuft. Das Verhältnis des Arztes zum Töten im allgemeinen und bedarf daher einer besonderen Erörterung.

Jeder Mensch ist bekanntlich unter gesetzlich näher bestimmten Umständen zu straflosen Eingriffen in fremde körperliche Existenz berechtigt (Notwehr, Notstand); beim Arzte wird das Verhältnis zum fremden Leben in negativer Hinsicht zwar durch das Gesetz bestimmt; tatsächlich ist aber sein Handeln auf diesem Gebiete ein Ausfluß seiner besonderen ärztlichen Sittenlehre. Es kommt der Allgemeinheit für gewöhnlich kaum zum Bewußtsein, daß diese ärztliche Sittenlehre nirgends fixiert ist. Es gibt wohl einzelne Bücher darüber, die aber den meisten Ärzten unbekannt sind und reine Privatleistungen ihrer Verfasser darstellen, aber es gibt kein in Paragraphen lebendes ärztliches Sittengesetz, keine "moralische Dienstanweisung"

Der junge Arzt geht ohne jede gesetzliche Umschreibung seiner Rechte und Pflichten gerade in bezug auf die eingreifenden Punkte in seine Praxis hinaus. Nicht einmal der Doktoreid der früheren Zeit mit einigen allgemeinen Bindungen ist mehr vorhanden. Was der Novize an Anweisung mitbringt, ist das Beispiel seiner Lehrer auf der Universität, die gelegentlichen Erörterungen, die sich an den Einzelfall anschlossen, das Lernen in seiner Assistentenzeit, der Einfluß der allgemeinen ärztlichen Anschauungen in der Literautr und eigene Schlußfolgerungen, die sich für ihn aus der Eigenart seiner Aufgabe ergeben. In gewissen Richtungen, aber gerade nicht in den entscheidenen, besteht eine Festlegung durch Gewerbeordnung, Verträge mit Krankenkassen u. dgl.; in einiger Entfernung sieht der Arzt einige Paragraphen des Strafgesetzbuches und die Aufsicht der Standesgenossen durch das ärztliche Ehrengericht. In allen diesen Punkten handelt es sich für den Arzt aber meist um eine negative Bindung in bezug auf das, was er nicht darf, nicht um positive Anweisungen. Was er darf und soll, ergibt sich als Ausfluß der Standesanschauungen, deren eine Voraussetzung unter allen Umständen die ist, daß der Arzt verpflichtet ist, nach allgemeinen sittlichen Normen zu handeln; dazu kommt als Standespflicht die Aufgabe, Kranke zu heilen, Schmerzen zu beseitigen oder zu lindern, Leben zu erhalten und soviel wie möglich, zu verlängern.

Diese allgemeine Regel ist nicht ohne Ausnahme. Der Arzt ist praktisch genötigt, Leben zu vernichten (Tötung des lebenden Kindes bei der Geburt im Interesse der Erhaltung der Mutter, Unterbrechung der Schwangerschaft aus gleichen Gründen). Diese Eingriffe sind nirgends ausdrücklich erblaubt; sie bleiben nur straflos von dem Gesichtspunkte aus, daß sie im Interesse der Sicherung eines höheren Rechtsgutes erfolgen und unter den Voraussetzungen, daß ihnen pflichtmäßige Erwägungen vorausgegangen sind, daß bei der Ausführung die Kunstregeln beachtet wurden, und daß die notwendige Verständigung mit dem Patienten oder seinem gesetzlichen Vertreter oder den Angehörigen stattgefunden hat.

Auch die Akte der Körperverletzung, wie sie der Chirurg berufsmäßig und spezialistisch vornimmt, sind nirgends ausdrücklich erlaubt. Sie bleiben nur straflos, wenn in bezug auf Prüfung der Notwendigkeit und Sorgfalt der Ausführung die Kunstregeln beachtet wurden. Dabei wird bei allen operativen Eingriffen stillschweigend auf einen gewissen Prozentsatz von tödlichen Ausgängen gerechnet, deren Herabdrückung auf das Mindestmaß das heißeste Bemühungen der ärztlichen Kunst ist, die aber niemals ganz ausbleiben können, wiederum also Fälle, in denen infolge ärztlicher Einwirkung Menschenleben vernichtet werden. Unser sittliches Gefühl hat sich hiermit völlig abgefunden. Das höhere Rechtsgut der Wiederherstellung einer Mehrzahl macht das Opfer einer Minderzahl notwendig, wobei im Einzelfalle die Sicherung in der Notwendigkeit der vorausgehenden Beschaffung der Einwilligung des Kranken oder seines gesetzlichen Vertreters im Eingriff gegeben ist, deren Voraussetzung in der Regel ist, daß ihm der Arzt nach bestem Wissen den Grad der Wahrscheinlichkeit der Wiederherstellung und auch der Lebensgefährdung auseinandergesetzt hat.

Auch außerhalb der oben genannten Arten von Fragen steht der Arzt häufig vor dem Problem eines Eingreifens in das Leben in sittlich zweifelhafter Situation. Von Angehörigen wird in Fällen unheilbarer Krankheit oder unheilbarer gesitiger Defektzustände nicht so selten der Wunsch geäußert, "daß es bald zu Ende sein möchte". Vor kurzem erst haben mich Angehörige einer in schwerer Bewußtlosigkeit liegenden Selbstmörderin, die das "schwarze Schaf" der Familie war, ersucht, doch ja nichts zur Wiederbelebung zu tun. Es kommt auch vor, daß die Familie im Affekt sich dazu versteigt, dem Arzte Vorwürfe zu machen, wenn der die aktive Verkürzung eines verlorenen evtl. schmerzensreichen Lebens ablehnt. Trotzdem ist von diesen gefühlsmäßigen Anwandlungen bis zu dem Entschlusse zur Tötung oder auch nur zu ausdrücklicher Einwilligung von seiten der Familie ein großer Schritt; wie die Menschen nun einmal sind, würde der Arzt, der heute selbst auf dringenden Wunsch der Angehörigen ein Leben verkürzte, in keiner Weise später vor den heftigen Vorwürfen oder auch vor einer Strafanzeige sicher sein.

Der Arzt kann gelegentlich auch in die Versuchung kommen, unter ganz bestimmten Umständen aus wissenschaftlichem Interesse in ein Menschenleben einzugreifen. Ich entsinne mich einer solchen Versuchung, die ich schließlich siegreich bestanden habe, aus meiner ersten Assistentenzeit. Ein Kind mit einer seltenen und wissenschaftliche interessanten Hirnerkrankung lag im Sterben, und der Zustand war so, daß mit Sicherheit im Laufe der nächsten 24 Stunden das Ende zu erwarten war. Wenn das Kind im Krankenhause starb, waren wir in der Lage, durch die Autopsie den erwünschten Einblick in den Befund zu erhalten. Nun erschien der Vater mit dem dringenden Verlangen, das Kind mit nach Hause zu nehmen; damit ging uns die Möglichkeit der Sektion verloren, die uns sicher war, wenn der Tod vor der Abholung eintrat. Es wäre ein Leichtes gewesen und hätte in keiner Weise festgestellt werden können, wenn ich damals durch eine Morphimeinspritzung den so wie so mit absoluter Sicherheit nahen Tod um einige Stunden verfrüht hätte. Ich habe schließlich doch nichts getan, weil mein persönlicher Wunsch nach wissenschaftlicher Erkenntnis mir kein genügend schwerwiegendes Rechtsgut sein durfte gegenüber der ärztlichen Pflicht, keine Lebensverkürzung vorzunehmen.

Wie man sich in einem solchen Falle zu entscheiden hätte, wenn etwa bei den geschilderten Umständen der Gewinn einer einschneidenden Einsicht mit der Wirkung späterer Rettung zahlreicher Menschenleben zu erwarten gewesen wäre, das wäre eine neue Frage, die von einem höheren Standpunkte aus mit Ja zu beantworten wäre.

In anderer Form streift das innere Dilemma den Arzt nicht so selten, wenn er vor der Frage steht, ob er durch passives Geschehenlassen, durch Unterlassen der entsprechenden Eingriffe, dem Tode freie Bahn öffnen soll in Fällen, in denen Kranke freiwillig das Leben zu verlassen wünschen und sich selbst in irgendeiner Form, auf dem Wege des Selbsttötungsversuches, in einen schwer gefährdeten Zustand versetzt haben.

Die Versuchung, in solchen Fällen dem Schicksal seinen Lauf zu lassen, ist dann besonders groß, wenn es sich etwa um unheilbare Geisteskranke handelt, bei denen der Tod das in jedem Falle Vorzuziehende ist.

(Selbstverständlich kann diese ganze Fragestellung dann nicht auftauchen, wenn es sich bei dem Kranken, wie etwa bei einer einfachen heilbaren Depression, um einen vorübergehenden Schätzungsirrtum in der Bewertung der zum Tode drängenden Motive gehandelt hat.)

Die kurze Aufzählung dieser Fälle, bei denen ich insgesamt aus eigener Erfahrung sprechen kann, zeigt, wie ungeheuer kompliziert schon im täglichen Leben sich für den Arzt die Abwägung zwischen den starren Grundsätzen der ärztlichen Norm und den Forderungen einer höheren Auffassung der Lebenswerte gestalten kann. Der Arzt hat kein absolutes, sondern nur ein relatives, unter neuen Umständen veränderliches, neu zu prüfendes Verhältnis zu der grundsätzlich anzuerkennenden Aufgabe der Erhaltung fremden Lebens unter allen Umständen. Die ärztliche Sittenlehre ist nicht als ein ewig gleichbleibendes Gebilde anzusehen. Die historische Entwicklung zeigt uns in dieser Hinsicht genügend deutliche Wandlungen. Von dem Augenblicke an, in dem z. B. die Tötung Unheilbarer oder die Beseitigung geistig Toter nicht nur als nicht strafbar, sondern als ein für die allgemeine Wohlfahrt wünschenswertes Ziel erkannt und allgemein anerkannt wäre, würden in der ärztlichen Sittenlehre jedenfalls keine ausschließenden Gegengründe zu finden sein.

Die Ärzte würden es z. B. zweifellos als eine Entlastung ihres Gewissens empfinden, wenn sie in ihrem Handeln an den Sterbebetten nicht mehr von dem kategorischen Gebote der unbedingten Lebens-verlängerung eingeengt und bedrückt würden, ein Gebot, zu dem ich mich auch - de lege lata - in meiner oben (S. 35) zitierten Äußerung bekannt habe; ich würde gern jenen Satz darin abändern dürfen: "es war früher eine unerläßliche Forderung..." Tatsächlich bedeuten die von Ärzten (oder auf ihre Anweisung vom Pflegepersonal und von den Angehörigen) vorgenommenen lebensverlängernden Eingriffe an Sterbenden für denjenigen, dem sie gelten und für den sie ein Gut darstellen sollen, vielfach ein Übel, eine Belästigung, eine Quälerei, in gleicher Weise wie für den gesunden, müden Einschlafenden die Störung durch immer wiederkehrende Weckreize; es liegt ihnen bei Laien in der weit überwiegenden Mehrzahl der Fälle eine falsche Vorstellung von dem inneren Zustande des Sterbenden zugrunde, dessen Bewußtsein entweder in heilsamer Weise verdunkelt ist, oder der nach langer Zermürbung durch Schmerzen und sonstiges Ungemach seiner Krankheit nur noch den Wunsch nach Ruhe und Schlafen hat und es sicherlich niemandem

Dank weiß, der sein immer tieferes Versinken in die Bewußtlosigkeit hindert und aufhält; er ist ja gar nicht mehr imstande, die gute Absicht hinter den störenden Pflegeeingriffen zu erkennen.

Das an sich anzuerkennende Prinzip der ärztlichen Pflicht zu möglichster Lebensverlängerung wird, auf die Spitze getrieben, zum Unsinn; "Wohltat wird zur Plage". Den Hauptgegenstand meiner ärztlichen Stellungnahme zu den rechtlichen Ausführungen soll die Beantwortung der oben Seite 28 formulierten Frage bilden: "Gibt es Menschenleben, die so stark die Eigenschaft des Rechtsguts eingebüßt haben, daß ihre Fortdauer für die Lebensträger wie für die Gesellschaft dauernd allen Wert verloren hat?"

Diese Frage ist im allgemeinen zunächst mit Bestimmtheit zu bejahen; im einzelnen ist dazu folgendes zu sagen. Die im juristischen Teile vollzogene Aufstellung der zwei Gruppen von hierhergehörigen Fällen entspricht den tatsächlichen Verhältnissen; der gemeinsame Gesichtspunkt des nicht mehr vorhandenen Lebenswertes faßt aber sehr Verschiedenartiges zusammen; bei der ersten Gruppe fder durch Krankheit oder Verwundung unrettbar Verlorenen wird nicht immer der subjektive und der objektive Lebenswert gleichmäßig aufgehoben sein, während bei der zweiten, auch zahlenmäßig größeren Gruppe der unheilbar Blödsinnigen, die Fortdauer des Lebens weder für die Gesellschaft noch für die Lebensträger selbst irgendwelchen Wert besitzt.

Zustände endgültigen unheilbaren Blödsinns oder wie wir in freundlicherer Formulierung sagen wollen: Zustände geistigen Todes sind für den Arzt, insbesondere für den Irrenarzt und Nervenarzt etwas recht Häufiges.

Man trennt sie zweckmäßigerweise in zwei große Gruppen:

1. in diejenigen Fälle, bei denen der geistige Tod im

späteren Verlaufe des Lebens nach vorausgehenden Zeiten geistiger Vollwertigkeit, oder wenigstens Durchschnittlichkeit erworben wird;

2. in diejenigen, die auf Grund angeborener oder in frühester Kindheit einsetzender Gehirnveränderungen entstehen.

Für die nicht ärztlichen Leser sei erwähnt, daß in der ersten Gruppe Zustände geistigen Todes erreicht werden: bei den Greisenveränderungen des Gehirns, dann bei der sogenannten Hirnerweichung der Laien, der Dementia paralytica, weiter auf Gund arteriosklerotischer Veränderungen im Gehirn und endlich bei der großen Gruppe der jugendlichen Verblödungsprozesse (Dementia praecox), von denen aber nur ein gewisser Prozentsatz die höchsten Grade geistiger Verblödung erreicht.

Bei der zweiten Gruppe handelt es sich entweder um grobe Mißbildungen des Gehirns, Fehlen einzelner Teile (in größerem oder geringerem Umfange), um Hemmungen der Entwicklung während der Eristenz im Mutterleib, die auch in die ersten Lebensjahre hinein weiter wirken knnen, oder um Krankheitsvorgänge der ersten Lebenszeit, die bei einem an sich normal angelegten Hirnorgan die Entwicklung sistieren; (häufig sind damit epileptische Anfälle oder andere motorische Reizerscheinungen verbunden).

Die beiden Gruppen können gleichhohe Grade der geistigen Ode vorhanden sein. Für unsere Zwecke aber ist doch ein Unterschied zu beachten, ein Unterschied in dem Zustande des geistigen Inventars, der vergleichsweise derselbe ist, wie zwischen einem regellos herumliegenden Haufen von Steinen, an die noch keine bildende Hand gerührt hat, und den Steintrümmern eines zusammengestürzten Gebäudes. Der Sachverständige vermag in der Regel, auch ohne Kenntnis der Vorgeschichte eines geistig toten Menschen und ohne körperliche Untersuchung aus der Art des geistigen Defektbildes die Unterscheidung der früh und der spät erworbenen Zustände zu machen.

Auch in den Beziehungen der zwei verschiedenen Arten geistig Toter zur Umwelt ist ein wesentlicher Unterschied für unsere Betrachtung vorhanden. Bei den ganz früh erworbenen hat niemals ein geistiger Rapport mit der Umgebung bestanden; bei den spät erworbenen ist dies vielleicht im rechten Maße der Fall gewesen. Die Umgebung, die Angehörigen und Freunde haben deswegen zu diesen letzteren subjektiv ein ganz anderes Verhältnis; geistig Tote dieser Art können einen ganz anderen "Affektionswert" erworben haben; ihnen gegenüber bestehen Gefühle der Pietät, der Dankbarkeit; zahlreiche, vielleicht stark gefühlsbetonte Erinnerungen verknüpfen sich mit ihrem Bilde, und alles dieses geschieht auch dann noch, wenn die Empfindungen der gesunden Umgebung bei dem Kranken keinerlei Widerhall mehr finden.

Aus diesem Grunde wird für die Frage der etwaigen Vernichtung nicht lebenswerter Leben aus der Reihe der geistig Toten, je nachdem sie der einen oder anderen Kategorie angehören, ein verschiedener Maßstab anzuwenden sein.

Auch in Bezug auf die wirtschaftliche und moralische Belastung der Umgebung, der Anstalten, des Staates usw. bedeuten die geistig Toten keineswegs immer das gleiche. Die geringste Belastung in dieser Richtung wird durch die Fälle von Hirnerweichung der einen oder anderen Art gegeben, die von dem Momente an, in welchem von geistigem völligem Tode gesprochen werden kann, in der Regel nur noch eine Lebensspanne von wenigen Jahren (höchstens) vor sich haben. Einen ein wenig weiteren Spielraum finden wir bei den Fällen von Greisenblödsinn. Die durch jugendlichen Prozesse geistig Verödeten können unter Umständen in diesem Zustande noch 20 oder 30 Jahre leben, während bei den Fällen von Vollidiotie auf Grund allerfrühester Veränderungen eine Lebensdauer und damit die Notwendigkeit fermder Führsorge von zwei Menschenaltern und darüber erwachsen kann.

In wirtschaftlicher Beziehung würden also diese Vollidioten, ebenso wie sie auch am ehesten alle Vorraussetzungen des vollständigen geistigen Todes erfüllen, gleichzeitig diejenigen sein, deren Existens am schwersten auf der Allgemeinheit lastet.

Diese Belastung ist zum Teil finanzieller Art und berechnbar an Hand der Aufstellung der Jahresbilanzen der Anstalten. Ich habe es mir angelegen sein lassen, durch eine Rundfrage bei sämtlichen deutschen in Frage kommenden Anstalten mir hierüber brauchbares Material zu verschaffen. Es ergibt sich daraus, daß der durchschnittliche Aufwand pro Kopf und Jahr für die Pflege der Idioten bisher 1300 M. betrug. Wenn wir die Zahl der in Deutschland zurzeit gleichzeitig vorhandenen, in Anstaltspflege befindlichen Idioten zusammenrechnen, so kommen wir schätzungsweise etwa auf eine Gesamtzahl von 20 - 30 000. Nehmen wir für den Einzelfall eine durchschnittliche Lebensdauer von 50 Jahren an, so ist leicht zu ermessen, welches ungeheure Kapital in Form von Nahrungsmitteln, Kleidung und Heizung, dem Nationalvermögen für einen unproduktiven Zweck entzogen wird.

Dabei ist hiermit noch keineswegs die wirkliche Belastung ausgedrückt.

Die Anstalten, die der Idiotenpflege dienen, werden anderen Zwecken entzogen; soweit es sich um Privatanstalten handelt, muß die Verzinsung berechnet werden; ein Pflegepersonal von vielen tausend Köpfenwird für diese gänzlich unfruchtbare Aufgabe festgelegt und fördernder Arbeit entzogen; es ist eine peinliche Vorstellung, daß ganze Generationen von Pflegern neben diesen leeren Menschenhülsen dahinaltern, von denen nicht wenige 70 Jahre und älter werden.

Die Frage, ob der für diese Kategorien von Ballastexistenzen notwendige Aufwand nach allen Richtungen hin gerechtfertigt sei, war in den verflossenen Zeiten des Wohlstandes nicht dringend; jetzt ist es anders geworden, und wir müssen uns ernstlich mit ihr beschäftigen. Unsere Lage ist wie die der Teilnehmer an einer schwierigen Expedition, bei welcher die größtmögliche Leistungsfähigkeit Aller die unerläßliche Voraussetzung für das Gelingen der Unternehmung bedeutet, und bei der kein Platz ist für halbe, Viertels und Achtels-Kräfte. Unsere deutsche Aufgabe wird für lange Zeit sein: eine bis zum höchsten gesteigerte Zusammenfassung aller Möglichkeiten, ein freimachen jeder verfügbaren Leistungsfähigkeit für fördernder Zwecke. Der Erfüllung dieser Aufgabe steht das moderne Bestreben entgegen, möglichst auch die Schwächlinge aller Sorten zu erhalten, allen, auch den zwar nicht geistig toten, aber doch ihrer Organisation nach minderewertigen Elemente Pflege und Schutz angedeihen zu lassen — Bemühungen, die dadurch ihre besondere Tragweite erhalten, daß es bisher nicht möglich gewesen, auch nicht im ernste versucht worden ist, diese von der Fortpflanzung auszuschließen.

Die ungeheure Schwierigkeit jedes Versuches, diesen Dingen irgendwie auf gesetzgeberischem Wege beizukommen, wird noch lange bestehen, und auch der gedanke, durch Freigabe der Vernichtung völlig wertloser, geistig Toter eine Entlastung für unsere nationale Überbürdung herbeizuführen, wird zunächst und vielleicht noch für weite Zeitstrecken lebhaftem, vorwiegend gefühlsmäßig vermitteltem Widerspruch begegnen, der seine Stärke aus sehr verschiedenen Quellen beziehen wird (Abneigung gegen das Neue, religiöse Bedenken, sentimentale Empfindungen usw.). In einer auf Erreichung möglichst greifbarer Ergebnisse gerichteten Untersuchung, wie der vorliegenden, soll daher dieser Punkt in der Form der theoretischen Erörterung der Möglichkeiten und Bedingungen, nicht aber in der des "Antrags" behandelt werden.

Bei allen Zuständen der Wertlosigkeit infolge geistigen Todes findet sich ein Widerspruch zwischen ihrem subjektiven Rechte auf Existenz und der objektiven Zweckmäßigkeit und Notwendigkeit.

Die Art der Lösung dieses Konfliktes war bisher der Maßstab für den Grad der in den einzelnen Menschheitsperioden und in den einzelnen Bezirken dieses Erdballs erreichten Humanität, zu deren heutigem Niveau ein langer mühsamer Entwicklungsgang über die Jahrtausende hin, zum Teil unter wesentlicher Mitwirkung christlicher Vorstellungsreihen, geführt hat.

Vor dem Standpunkte einer höheren staatlichen Sittlichkeit aus gesehen kann nicht wohl bezweifelt werden, daß in dem Streben nach unbedingter Erhaltung lebensunwerter Leben Übertreibungen geübt worden sind. Wir haben es, von fremden Gesichtspunkten aus, verlernt, in dieser Beziehung den staatlichen Organismus im selben Sinne wie ein Ganzes mit eigenen Gesetzen und Rechten zu betrachten, wie ihn etwa ein in sich geschlossener menschlicher Organismus darstellt, der wie wir Ärzte wissen, im Inreresse der Wohlfahrt des Ganzen auch einzelne werlos gewordene oder schädliche Teile oder Teilchen preisgibt und abstößt.

Ein Überblick über die oben aufgestellte Reihe der Ballastexistenzen und ein kurzes Nachdenken zeigt, daß die Mehrzahl davon für die Frage einer Bewußten Abstoßung, d.h. Beseitigung nicht in Betracht kommt. Wir weden auch in den Zeiten der Not, dennen entgegengehen, nie aufhören wollen, Defekte und Sieche zu pflegen, solange sie nicht geistig tot sind; wir werden nie aufhören, körperlich und geistig Erkrankte bis zum Äußertsten zu behandeln, solange noch irgendeine Aussicht auf Änderung ihres Zustandes zum Guten vorhanden ist; aber wir weden vielleicht eines Tages zu der Auffassung herranreifen, daß die *Beseitigung der Geistig völlig Toten kein Verbrechen, keine unmoralische Handlung, keine gefühlsmäßige Rohheit, sondern einen erlaubten nützlichen Akt darstellt.*

Hier intressiert uns nun zunächst die Frage, welche Eigenschaften und Wirkungen den Zuständen geistigen Todes zukommen. In äußerlicher Beziehung ist ohne weiteres erkennbar: der Fremdkörpercharakter der geistig Toten im Gefüge der menschlichen Gesellschaft, das fehlen irgendwelcher produktiver Leistungen, einZustand völliger Hilflosigkeit mit der Notwendigkeit der Versorgung durch Dritte.

In bezug auf den inneren Zustand würde zum Begriff des geistigen Todes gehören, daß nach der Art der Hirnbeschaffenheit klare Vorstellungen, Gefühle oder Willensregungen nicht entstehen können, daß keine Möglichkeit der Erweckung eines Weltbildes im Bewußtsein besteht, und das keine Gefühlsbeziehungen zur Umwelt von den geistig Toten ausgehen können, (wenn sie auch natürlich Gegenstand der Zuneigung von seiten Dritter sein mögen).

Das Wesendlichste aber ist das Fehlen der Möglichkeit, sich der eigenen Persöhnlichkeit bewußt zu werden, das Fehlen des Selbstbewußtseins. Die geistig Toten stehen auf einem intellektuellen Niveau, das wir erst tief unten in der tierreihe wieder finden, und auch die Gefühlsregungen erheben sich nicht über die Linie elementarster, an das animalische Leben gebundener Vorgänge.

Ein geistig Toter ist somit auch nicht imstande, innerlich einen subjektiven Anspruch auf Leben erheben zu Können, ebensowenig wie er anderer geistiger Prozesse fähig wäre.

Dieses letztere ist nur scheinbar unwesentlich; in Wirklichkeit hat es seine Bedeutung in dem Sinne, daß die Beseitigung eines geistig Toten einer sonstigen Tötung nicht gleichzusetzen ist. Schon rein juristisch bedeutet die Vernichtung eines Menschenlebens keineswegs immer dasselbe.

Die Unterschiede liegen nicht nur in den Motiven

des Tötenden, (je nachdem: Mord, Totschlag, Fahrlässigkeit, Notwehr, Zweikampf usw.), sondern auch in dem Verhältnis des Getöteten zu seinem Anspruch auf Leben. Während die vorsätzliche überlegte Tötung gegen den Willen eines Menschen die Todesstrafe nach sich zieht, wird die Tötung auf Verlangen nur mit ein paar Jahren Gefängnis geahndet. Der Akt des Eingreifens in fremdes Leben ist dabei jedesmal derselbe. Die Tötung auf Verlangen wird dabei im Zweifelsfalle eher noch eine kühlere, planmäßigere, reiflicher überlegte Handlung bedeuten, als der Mord, und doch wird sie unter anderem darum so viel milder aufgefaßt, weil der zu Tötende sich seines subjektiven Anspruches auf das Leben begeben hat, und im Gegenteil sein Recht auf den Tod geltend macht.

(An dieser Betrachtung ändert sich dadurch nichts, daß es auch heilbare Geisteskranke gibt, die keinen subjektiven Anspruch auf Leben, im Gegenteil sogar energischen Anspruch auf die Vernichtung machen, die aber weil es sich um krankhafte Motive episodischer Art handelt, in ihrem Wollen überhaupt keine Berücksichtigung verdienen; diese Fälle sind übrigens von dem Zustande des geistigen Todes weit entfernt.)

Im Falle der Tötung eines geistig Toten, der nach Lage der Dinge, vermöge seines Hirnzustandes, nicht imstande ist, subjektiven Anspruch auf irgend etwas, u.a. also auch auf das Leben zu erheben, wird somit auch kein subjektiver Anspruch verletzt.

Es ergibt sich aus dem, was über den inneren geistigen Zustand der geistig Toten zu sagen war, auch ohne weiteres das es falsch ist, ihnen gegenüber den Gesichtspunkt des Mitleids geltend zu machen; es liegt dem Mitleid mit den lebensunwerten Leben der unausrottbare Denkfehler oder besser Denkmangel zugrunde, vermöge dessen die Mehrzahl der Menschen in fremde lebende Gebilde hinein ihr eigenes Denken und Fühlen projiziert, ein Irrtum, der auch eine der Quellen der

Auswüchse des Tierkultus beim europäischen Menschen darstellt. " Mitleid" ist den geistig Toten gegenüber im Leben und im Sterbensfall die an letzter Stelle angebrachte Gefühlsregung; Wo kein Leiden ist, ist auch kein mitLeiden.

Trotz alledem wird in dieser neuen Frage nur ein ganz langsam sich entwickelnder Prozeß der Umstellung und Neueinstellung möglich sein. Das Bewußtsein der Bedeutungslosigkeit der Einzelexistenz, gemessen an den Interessen des Ganzen, das Gefühl einer absoluten Verpflichtung zur Zusammenraffung aller verfügbaren Kräfte unter Abstoßung aller unnötigen Aufgaben, das Gefühl, höchst verantwortlicher Teilnehmer einer schweren und leidensvollen Unternehmung zu sein , wird in viel höherem Maße, als heute, Allgemeinbesitz werden müssen, ehe die hier ausgesprochenen Anschauungen volle Anerkennung finden können. Die Menschen sind im allgemeinen großer und starker Gefühle nur ausnahmsweise und immer nur für kurze Zeit fähig; deswegen machen besondere Einzelbetätigungen in dieser Richtung einen so großen Eindruck. Wir lesen mit tragischem Mitgefühl in Greelys Polarbericht, wie er genötigt ist, um die Lebenswahrscheinlichkeit der Teilnehmer zu erhöhen, einen der Genossen, der sich an die Rationierung nicht hielt und durch unerlaubtes Essen eine Gefahr für alle wurde, von hinten erschießen zu lassen, da er ihnen allen an Körperkräften überlegen geworden war; ein berechtigtes Mitleid überkommt uns, wenn wir lesen, wie Kapt. Scott und seine Begleiter auf der Heimkehr vom Südpol im Interesse des Lebens der Übrigen schweigend das Opfer annahm, daß ein Teilnehmer freiwillig das Zelt verließ, um draußen im Schnee zu erfrieren.

Ein kleiner Teil solcher heroischen Seelenstimmungen müßte uns beschieden sein, ehe wir an die Verwirklichung der hier theoretisch erörterten Möglichkeiten herantreten können.

Sache der ärztlichen Beurteilung ist schließlich alles, was sich in dem Zusammenhange unserer Darstellung auf die Notwendigkeit technischer Sicherungen gegen irrtümliches oder mißbräuchliches Vorgehen bezieht.

Zunächst wird selbstverständlich die Idee auftauchen, daß die Verwirklichung der hier ausgesprochenen Gedanken krimminellen Mißbräuchen die Tür öffnen könnte. Vermöge des ständig wachen Mißtrauens, das der normale Staaatsbürger vielfach gesetzgeberischen Dingen entgegenbringt, die irgendwie in seine private Existenz eingreifen, werden auch hier möglichkeiten gewittert und ins Feld geführt werden. Es liegt dem dieselbe Richtung des Fühlens und Denkens zugrunde, die mühelos dazu kommt, anzunehmen, daß es für Wohlhabende eine Kleinigkeit sei, sich vermöge ärztlicher Atteste in Straffällen ihre Unzurechnungsfähigkeit bekunden zu lassen, die es dem Laien durchaus glaubhaft und wahrscheinlich macht, daß fortwährend internierungen geistig Gesunder und Entmündigungen aus gwinnsüchtigen Motiven der Angehörigen erfolgen, Anschauungen, die sich sogar zu der gesetzgeberischen praktischen Unzweckmäßigkeit verdichtet haben, daß in der Entmündigungsfrage das Antragsrecht des Staatsanwaltes seinerzeit eingeschränkt worden ist (bei Trunksucht).

Die Sicherung gegen solche Auffassungen würde in einer sorgfältig zu behandelnden Technik zu schaffen sein.

In dieser Beziehung steht zunächst zur Erörterung, ob die Auswahl der Fälle, die für die Lebensträger selbst und für die Gesellschaft endgültig wertlos geworden sind, mit solcher Sicherheit getroffen werden kann, daß Fehlgriffe und Irrtümer ausgeschlossen sind.

Es kann dies nur eines Laien Sorge sein. Für den Arzt besteht nicht der geringste Zweifel, daß diese Auswahl mit hundertprozentiger Sicherheit zu treffen ist, also mit einem ganz anderen Maße von Sicherheit, als etwa bei hinzurichtenden Verbrechern die Frage, ob sie geistig gesund , oder geistig krank sind, entschieden werden kann.

Für den Arzt bestehen zahlreiche wissenschaftliche, keiner Diskussion mehr unterworfene Kriterien, aus denen die Unmöglichkeit der Besserung eines geistig Toten erkannt werden kann, um so mehr, als für unsere ganze Fragestellung in vorderster Linie die frühere Jugend an bestehenden Zustände geistigen Todes in Betracht kommen.

Natürlich wird kein Arzt schon bei einem Kinde im zweiten oder dritten Lebensjahr die Sicherheit dauernden geistigen Todes behaupten wollen. Es kommt aber noch in der Kindheit der Momment, in dem auch diese Zukunftsbestimmung zweifelsfrei getroffen werden kann.

Es ist in dem juristischem Teil dieser Schrift schon die Art der Zusammensetzung einer zur genauesten Prüfung der Lage berufenen Kommission besprochen worden. Auch ich bin überzeugt, daß trotz des Beiklanges von Fruchtlosigkeit, den wir bei der Erwähnung des Wortes " Kommission" innerlich hören, eine derartige Einrichtung notwendig sein würde. Die Erörterung der Einzelheiten halte ich für weniger dringend, als das Bekenntnis dazu, daß selbstverständlich die Voraussetzung für die Verwirklichung dieser Gedankengänge die Schaffung aller denkbaren Garantien nach jeder Richtung sein muß.

Von Goehte stammt das Bild des Entwicklungsganges wichtiger Menschheitsfragen, den er sich in Spiralform versinnlicht. Die Achse dieses Bildes ist die Tatsache, daß eine etwa an einem Stamme emporlaufende Spirallinie in gewissen Abständen immer wieder auf derselben Seite des Stammes ankommt und vorüberführt, aber jedesmal ein Stockwerk höher.

Dieses Bild wird sich später auch in dieser unserer

Kulturfrage erkennen lassen. Es gab eine Zeit, die wir jetzt als barbarisch betrachten, in der die Beseitigung der lebensunfähig Geborenen selbstverständlich war, dann kam die jetzt noch laufende Phase, in welcher schließlich die Erhaltung jeder noch so wertlosenExistenz als höchste sittliche Forderung galt; eine neue Zeit wird kommen, die von dem Standpunkte einer höheren Sittlichkeit aus aufhören wird, die Forderung eines überspannten Humanitätsbegriffes und einer Überschätzung des Wertes der Existenz schlechthin mit schweren Opfern dauernd in die Tat umzusetzen. Ich weiß, daß diese Ausführungenheute keineswegs überall schon Zustimmung oder auch nur Verständnis finden werden; dieser Gesichtspunkt darf Denjenigen nicht zum Schweigen Veranlassen, der nach mehr als einem Menschenalter ärztlichen Menschendienstes das Recht beanspruchen kann, in allgemeinen Menschheitsfragen gehört zu werden.

Printed in the USA
CPSIA information can be obtained
at www.ICGtesting.com
LVHW071345140923
757947LV00001B/120